Baby & Child Medical Care

The Meadowbrook Medical Reference Group

Edited by Mitchell J. Einzig, M.D., and
Terril H. Hart, M.D.

Meadowbrook Press
Distributed by Simon & Schuster
New York

Library of Congress Cataloging-in-Publication Data

Baby & child medical care / the Meadowbrook Medical Reference Group : edited by Mitchell J.
    Einzig and Terril H. Hart. — [3rd ed.]
        p.   cm.
    Rev. ed. of : The Parent's guide to baby & child medical care. c1991.
    ISBN 0-88166-307-7 (Meadowbrook)
    ISBN 0-671-58000-0 (Simon & Schuster)
    1. Pediatrics—Popular works. 2. Children—Diseases. I. Einzig, Mitchell J. II. Hart, Terril H.,
    1939- . III. Meadowbrook Medical Reference Group. IV. Parent's guide to baby & child
    medical care.
    RJ61.P2245 1998
    618.92—dc21   97-36441
                                                                         CIP

Medical Editors: Mitchell J. Einzig, M.D., and Terril H. Hart, M.D.
Coordinating Editor (1997 revision): Liya Lev Oertel
Copyeditor (1997 revision): Nancy Baldrica
Production Manager: Joe Gagne
Production Assistant: Danielle White
Illustrator: Nancy Lynch

Portions of the text of this book appeared originally in *The Family Doctor's Health Tips* by Keith
W. Sehnert, M.D. They are reprinted herein with permission.

The editors thank American Heart Association instructor/trainer Carole Shea, R.N., for
reviewing the Breathing Emergency, Cardiac Arrest, and Choking step-by-step treatments.

The contents of this book have been reviewed and checked for accuracy and appropriateness of
application by medical doctors. However, the editors and publisher disclaim all responsibility
arising from any adverse effects or results which occur or might occur as a result of the
inappropriate application of any of the information contained in this book. If you have any
question or concern about the appropriateness or application of the treatments described in
this book, consult your health-care professional.

Published by Meadowbrook Press, 5451 Smetana Drive, Minnetonka, MN 55343

BOOK TRADE DISTRIBUTION by Simon & Schuster, a division of Simon and Schuster, Inc.,
1230 Avenue of the Americas, New York, NY 10020

First Published in the UK 1991

DISTRIBUTION IN THE UK AND IRELAND by Chris Lloyd Sales and Marketing, P.O. Box 327,
Poole, Dorset BH15 2RG

02 01 00 99 98   18 17 16 15 14 13 12 11 10 9 8

Printed in the United States of America

CONTENTS

Part One: Keeping Your Child Healthy

Part Two: Helping Your Child Get Better

Part Three: Step-by-Step Treatments

Part Four: Appendix

Charts and Tables

INTRODUCTION

New discoveries and changes are constantly occuring in the field of medicine, thus information becomes obsolete almost as soon as it is published. Why, then, the continued popularity of *Baby & Child Medical Care*? Since its publication, hundreds of thousands of families have come to rely upon it to help them respond effectively to their children's illnesses and injuries.

Perhaps parents keep turning to *Baby & Child Medical Care* because the book focuses on easy use, clear writing, and rigorous accuracy, giving parents confidence to better take care of their children. *Baby & Child Medical Care*'s reader-friendly design will enable you to tell at a glance whether to contact professional help or treat the problem at home using the clearly laid out numbered or bulleted instructions and illustrations.

Now, with this all-new Third Edition, the lead editorship has passed to the expert care of Mitchell J. Einzig, M.D., whose skills as a pediatrician, educator, and writer have brought this book to a new level of excellence and usefulness. Between the two of us we bring over fifty years of the practice of pediatrics to this volume. I hope that it contributes to improved health for children and their families everywhere.

Dr. Einzig and I dedicate this Third Edition to the staff, past and present, of the Wayzata Children's Clinic.

Terril H. Hart, M.D.

PART ONE

Keeping Your Child Healthy

Raising happy, healthy children presents parents with daily challenges. Effectively meeting these challenges requires calm, self-confident parents who understand their child's uniqueness. Remember, *you* are the expert when it comes to your child. This book will provide information to help you care for your child, whether sick or well, so you can meet the daily challenges head on! A caring, self-confident parent and a happy, healthy child with a high level of self-esteem go hand-in-hand.

Choosing a Doctor

The first step in maintaining your child's health is choosing a health care professional. The partnership between you, your child, and your doctor extends from the prenatal period through adolescence. Your doctor will also provide guidance through the ups and downs of childrearing. Below are some things to consider when choosing a doctor.

Personal Qualities of Your Doctor:
The health care professional you choose should
- care about you and your child and relate well to both of you.
- have effective communication skills.
- listen to your concerns and questions.

Your Personal Expectations:
You should decide whether you prefer
- a male or female doctor.
- a pediatrician—a doctor who has three or more years of

postmedical school training specifically in child and adolescent health, or
- a family physician—a doctor who has three years of postmedical school training in all areas of medicine, and who will likely care for both you and your children.

Your Professional Expectations:

When choosing a doctor, remember the following:
- Your doctor is not infallible.
- Your doctor may not be able to make an exact diagnosis if your child has had symptoms for only a brief period. Often, follow-up calls or visits are important to clarify the diagnosis.
- Your doctor may not always prescribe treatment with an antibiotic or other medicine. If a viral infection is diagnosed, no prescription or over-the-counter medication may be indicated. You must remember that many symptoms represent the body's defenses against infection. For example, coughs help clear secretions from the windpipe and bronchial tubes. Vomiting may be a way for the body to rid itself of infectious organisms or toxins.

Always ask why your doctor is prescribing an antibiotic, not why he or she is not prescribing one. In the past few years, some bacteria have become resistant to many or all of the currently available antibiotics. In the antibiotic war against infectious diseases, the "bugs" seem to be getting the upper hand. In part, this is due to the unnecessary use of antibiotics. Parents should remember that the majority of childhood infections are caused by viruses and do not require antibiotic treatment.

Professional Qualities of the Doctor's Office:

- Pediatric nurse practitioners, physician assistants, and other health professionals may play a role in your child's health care. They should be knowledgeable, professional, and helpful.
- All office staff should be friendly and courteous and treat you and your child with respect.
- Office visits should be efficient, and waits should not be unduly long.

Finding a Doctor

Many health care organizations offer referral services to help you find a doctor. Other ways to locate a doctor include the following:
- tips from friends
- referrals from your obstetrician or physician
- recommendations from the local hospital or your other doctors.
- personal interviews (These are especially important in the prenatal period.)

If You Are Not Happy with Your Choice
- Discuss your concerns with your doctor. He or she may not be aware of what you perceive as a problem.
- Change doctors if problems persist. The relationship with the doctor you choose may very well last for many years. You should be comfortable with and confident in your doctor.
- If you decide to switch doctors, schedule an introductory visit to evaluate your new doctor.

Health Supervision

Regular health supervision or doctor office visits provide you and your doctor opportunities to
- Monitor your child's growth and development. At each visit, your physician will plot your child's progress with respect to height, weight, and head growth. Some offices will perform a Denver Developmental Standardized Test (DDST). This simple office test, often done by a nurse, assesses the child's personal/social, speech, fine motor, and gross motor development. DDST is not an intelligence test.
- Discuss your concerns and answer questions. Each of your child's developmental stages brings new challenges and concerns.
- Perform a physical examination.
- Provide immunizations ("shots").
- Perform various screening tests (hearing, vision, and so on).
- Provide anticipatory guidance—information about the next stage of development. This information is designed to help you improve your parenting skills for the challenges ahead. In providing anticipatory guidance, your doctor should discuss child behavior, some of the unique characteristics of the next developmental stage, injury prevention, nutrition, and oral health. Brochures or handouts may be provided to help you adapt to the forthcoming changes.

Checklist for Choosing a Doctor

The following checklist should help you identify and narrow down your choices.

Basic Information

Name _____

Address _____

Phone (office)_____ (pager) _____

      (24-hour answering service) _____

      Fax _____

Hospital affiliation(s) _____

Type of Professionals in Office
___ pediatrician or   ___ family practitioner
___ board certified or   ___ board eligible
___ pediatric nurse-practitioner
___ physician's assistant (P.A.)

Type of Practice
___ solo practice   ___ small group   ___large group
                          practice   practice

Professional Affiliations (check one or more)
___ teaching appointment at a university
___ on staff at hospital of your choice
___ member of professional medical group(s)

Services
___ sees patients by appointment only
___ allows walk-in visits
___ practice covered at all times
___ allows at least 15–20 minutes for each health supervision visit
___ conducts a thorough baseline history
___ medical records available if requested (always open to patient)
___ gives advice on the phone (24-hour phone availability)

Accessibility
___ bus or nearby public transportation
___ wheelchair accessible
___ wheelchair available
___ free parking nearby

Additional Services
___ waiting area child friendly
___ baby-sitting
___ patient-education classes/material available in waiting area
___ patient-advocate services
___ interpreter (for languages other than English, or for hearing impaired)

Medical/Laboratory Services
___ X-ray in building or nearby
___ minor surgery in office
___ blood tests
___ casting and minor orthopedic services
___ generic medications optional on prescriptions

Billing Information
___ immediate payment required
___ new patient prepayment required
___ accepts Medicaid
___ will discuss fees and charges
___ will help prepare insurance forms
___ accept credit cards
___ discount for immediate cash payments

Medical Philosophy
The professional's positions on:

vitamins and nutrition _____

medical self-care _____

antibiotics _____

circumcision _____

breastfeeding _____

second opinions _____

other issues _____

_____

_____

_____

_____

Health Screenings and Assessments for Children Ages Birth to 2 Years
Recommendations of the American Academy of Pediatrics (AAP)

(These are recommendations; variations may be appropriate based on your child's history and your physician's assessment.)

	INFANCY						CHILDHOOD			
	by 2-3 days	1 mo	2 mo	4 mo	6 mo	9 mo	12 mo	15 mo	18 mo	24 mo
Medical History/ Interview (Health Profile)	•	•	•	•	•	•	•	•	•	•
Measurements										
Height/Weight	•	•	•	•	•	•	•	•	•	•
Head Circumference	•	•	•	•	•	•	•	•	•	•
Tests/Screenings										
Vision	•	•	•	•	•	•	•	•	•	•
Hearing	•	•	•	•	•	•	•	•	•	•
Blood Pressure										
Blood Tests[1]										
Urinalysis[1]										
Heredity/Metabolic	•									
Hemoglobin[3]										
Tuberculin[4]										
Development/ Behavior Assessment	•	•	•	•	•	•	•	•	•	•
Physical Examination	•	•	•	•	•	•	•	•	•	•
Dental Checkup[2]							•			
Anticipatory Guidance	•	•	•	•	•	•	•	•	•	•

[1]At least once during infancy, early childhood, late childhood, and adolescence.
[2]Initial dental referral at 12-18 months. Initial visit at 2½-3 years and every 6 months thereafter.
[3]At 6-12 months for high-risk infants only.
[4]In high-risk populations only.

Health Screenings and Assessments for Children Ages 3 to 18 Years
Recommendations of the American Academy of Pediatrics (AAP)

(These are recommendations; variations may be appropriate based on your child's history and your physician's assessment.)

	CHILDHOOD					ADOLESCENCE				
	3 yrs	4 yrs	5 yrs	6 yrs	8 yrs	10 yrs	12 yrs	14 yrs	16 yrs	18 yrs
Medical History/ Interview (Health Profile)	•	•	•	•	•	•	•	•	•	•
Measurements										
Height/Weight	•	•	•	•	•	•	•	•	•	•
Head Circumference										
Tests/Screenings										
Vision	•	•	•	•	•	•	•	•	•	•
Hearing	•	•	•	•	•	•	•	•	•	•
Blood Pressure	•	•	•	•	•	•	•	•	•	•
Blood Tests[1]										
Urinalysis[1]										
Heredity/Metabolic										
Hemoglobin[3]										
Tuberculin[4]										
Development/ Behavior Assessment	•	•	•	•	•	•	•	•	•	•
Physical Examination	•	•		•	•	•	•	•	•	•
Dental Checkup[2]										
Anticipatory Guidance	•	•	•	•	•	•	•	•	•	•

[1]At least once during infancy, early childhood, late childhood, and adolescence.
[2]Initial dental referral at 12-18 months. Initial visit at 2½-3 years and every 6 months thereafter.
[3]At 6-12 months for high-risk infants only.
[4]In high-risk populations only.

Immunizations

Immunizations (or shots) protect your child against many serious life-threatening infectious diseases. For this reason, it is very important for your child to receive all immunizations at the recommended time. Newer vaccines, such as the Chicken Pox vaccine and various combination vaccines, are being added to the routine schedule each year.

Recommended Immunizations
for Children Ages Birth through 16 Years

Approved by the Advisory Committee on Immunization Practices (ACIP), the American Academy of Pediatrics (AAP), and the American Academy of Family Physicians (AAFP)

(With the advent of new vaccines and new vaccine combinations, this schedule is subject to change. This schedule is the recommended schedule for January through December 1998. Ranges indicate acceptable ages for vaccination. Recognized abbreviations follow in parenthesis.)

Birth–2 Months
Hepatitis B-1 (Hep B-1)

1–4 Months
Hepatitis B-2 (Hep B-2)

2 Months
Hepatitis B-1 (Hep B-1), *if not received earlier than age 2 months*
Diphtheria, Tetanus, Pertussis (DTaP or DTP)
H. influenzae type b (Hib)
Polio

4 Months
Hepatitis B-2 (Hep B-2), *if not received earlier than age 4 months*
Diphtheria, Tetanus, Pertussis (DTaP or DTP)
H. influenzae type b (Hib)
Polio

6 Months
Diphtheria, Tetanus, Pertussis (DTaP or DTP)
H. influenzae type b (Hib)

6–18 Months
Hepatitis B-3 (Hep B-3)
Polio

12–15 Months
H. influenzae type b (Hib)
Measles, Mumps, Rubella (MMR)

12–18 Months
Varicella (Chicken Pox)

15–18 Months
Diphtheria, Tetanus, Pertussis (DTaP or DTP)

4–6 Years
Diphtheria, Tetanus, Pertussis (DTaP or DTP)
Polio
Measles, Mumps, Rubella (MMR), *or may be given between ages 11–12*

11–12 Years
Hep B, *given at this age as a catch-up vaccination to those children not previously vaccinated.*
Measles, Mumps, Rubella (MMR), *if not given between ages 4–6.*
Varicella (Var), *given at this age as a catch-up vaccination to those children not previously vaccinated.*

11–16 Years
Tetanus and Diphtheria toxoids (Td), *recommended if at least 5 years have elapsed since the last dose of DTP, DTaP, or DT. Routine Td boosters are recommended every 10 years.*

Injury Prevention:
Child Safety Is No Accident

As children grow, so do their abilities. In a matter of days, an infant can learn to walk; a toddler can learn to climb. Between the ages of 1 and 2, your child will learn to walk, run, climb, jump, and explore. Between the ages 2 and 4, your child will learn new skills, quickly. She will now move more confidently, ride a tricycle, and use tools. And while these abilities are exciting, they can also lead to serious problems—if you are not prepared.

In the United States, injuries are responsible for more deaths among children and teenagers than all diseases combined. Each year, 30,000 American children suffer permanent disability from injuries, and one in five are injured seriously enough to require medical care. The American Academy of Pediatrics (AAP) developed TIPP—The Injury Prevention Program—a few years ago. This program includes a specific safety counseling schedule that discusses age-appropriate safety devices and offers age-appropriate safety take-home sheets that your health care professional can provide.

The three most common causes of serious childhood injuries involve automobiles, drowning, and home fires. The following suggestions will help you prevent injuries due to these causes, as well as injuries due to falls, kitchen accidents, and poisons.

The information below was compiled from the American Academy of Pediatrics TIPP guidelines. It is designed to help you understand your child's special abilities from ages 1 to 4, so you can make your home a safe place for your child to grow.

Automobile Safety

More children are killed in auto accidents than in any other way. Yet, almost all these deaths are preventable. In most states, proper seat restraints are required by law. Your insistence upon their use will ensure your child's safety. And remember: NEVER place an infant—either front-facing or rear-facing—in the front seat of a vehicle with passenger-side airbags. Infants and children have been seriously injured and killed as a result of airbag inflation during collision.

Intervention
- Use child safety seats. Safety seats reduce the likelihood of fatal injuries by 70 percent.
- Never put an infant in the front seat of a car with a passenger-side air bag. If your child must ride in the front seat in an

emergency, move the seat as far back—away from the air bag—as possible.

- Place your infant and child (through school age) in the back seat of your car. That is the safest place to ride.
- Use a rear-facing infant seat in the back seat for children from birth to 20 lbs.
- Use a convertible seat for infants from birth to 40 lbs. Infants under 20 lbs. should use rear-facing seats; infants over 20 lbs. should use forward-facing seats.
- Use booster seats:
  —Children over 30 lbs. should use the belt-position type.
  —Children 40–65 lbs. should use the shield type (if only a lap belt is available).
  —Children over 40 lbs. (age 4–5) should sit straight up against the back seat, on a cushion, with the belt across their hips.
- Use seat belts alone when your child's ears extend above the rear of the back seat.
- Always follow manufacturers' instructions regarding car-seat usage and maintenance.
- Encourage your child to ride quietly in the car, so you will not be distracted.

Drowning

Drowning is second only to motor-vehicle-occupant injury as a cause of death for children ages birth-14 years. Young children drown primarily at home (pools, bathtubs, water pails). Older children tend to drown in recreational mishaps (boating, swimming in unsupervised areas).

Intervention

- Have constant adult supervision for children in or near water:
  —Maintain constant eye contact with nonswimmers in pool environments.
  —Require that supervising adults be trained in CPR. Check with your doctor, fire station, school, or hospital about classes.
  —Keep a telephone by the pool, in case of emergency.
- Surround pools with 5-foot fencing and a self-closing and self-latching gate. Cover pools when not in use.
- Offer children swimming lessons. There is ongoing debate about the value of swimming lessons for infants under one year of age. The American Academy of Pediatrics recommends against organized swimming instruction before age 3. It is unlikely that infants can be made "water safe." Children

younger than 3 can be taught to come to the surface, float, and paddle, but whether a child can retain and apply this information in emergency situations is debatable.

Home Fires
There's been a recent decrease in home fires due to the increased use of smoke detectors. This has reduced the risk of dying in a fire by 50 percent.

Intervention
- Test smoke detectors once a month, and change batteries once a year. To help you remember to check your detectors, schedule maintenance to coincide with one of your children's birthdays or with Daylight Savings clock changes.
- Discourage the use of portable heaters, especially at night.
- Buy only flame-resistant sleepwear for your child (pure cotton is not flame-resistant).

Poisons
Nine out of ten poisonings occur in the home. Your child cannot read or distinguish potentially harmful substances by taste or smell alone. Therefore, he depends on you to keep his environment safe and free of poisons. Here are some suggestions to get you started. (Remember: Homes you visit may not be childproofed. Look for potentially harmful substances your child may encounter in new locations.)

Intervention
- Make sure that all potentially harmful products come in child-resistant packaging.
- Read all product and medication labels, and follow medication dosage recommendations.
- Place poison warning stickers, such as "Mr. Yuk," on poisonous substances. Mr. Yuk's* expression conveys the idea that the substance will taste bad—something a child will understand better than the possibility of death. (You can get these stickers for a dollar from the Poison Center, 1 Children's Place, 3705 5th Ave. at DeSoto, Pittsburgh, PA 5213.) Caution: Do not place excessive confidence in this measure alone; keep poisonous substances LOCKED UP.

*Mr. Yuk, the poison warning symbol of the Poison Center, Pittsburgh

- Keep all household products in their original containers, and do not store these substances near food.
- Store poisonous substances in "safe" locations—out of children's reach and secured with child-resistant safety locks.
- Post the phone number of the regional Poison Information Center by your telephone.
- Keep a 1-ounce bottle of syrup of ipecac at home and in the car glove compartment to induce vomiting when indicated.
- Have your pharmacist dispense all medicines with safety closures, don't take your own medicine in front of young children and toddlers, and never give your child's medication to another child.
- Flush leftover medication down the toilet.
- Get rid of leftover alcoholic beverages immediately after a party.
- Remove any poisonous plants from your yard. Know whether your houseplants are poisonous.

If your child ingests poison, do not panic: Call your local poison center or dial 911
You will be asked to
- identify yourself, your child, and your child's age and weight;
- identify the poison or medication your child has ingested;
- estimate how much poison your child ingested and when;
- describe any first-aid measures you have taken.

Time is of the essence. Call your poison control center or emergency number (911) if you even suspect your child has ingested a poisonous substance. Emergency personnel will tell you what actions to take.

When you take your child to an emergency facility,
- Bring the poison, pills, plants, containers, or other substance your child has ingested.
- Supply a sample of vomit. (Do not induce vomiting unless instructed to do so.)
- Do not attempt any first aid unless instructed to do so.

Falls
The risk of falls grows as your child grows. "Toddlers" is more than just a name for children ages 1 to 2. It accurately describes how they move. Children in this age group are prone to fall and seriously injure themselves on sharp furniture edges or while riding

their bikes. Chairs allow them access to higher ground. Stairs can pose hazardous obstacles. Baby walkers can be especially dangerous near stairs. As children grow, they can climb onto, and therefore fall off, higher places. Anything your child can climb can be dangerous: playground equipment, beds, windows, and so on.

Intervention
- Use gates on stairs.
- Secure windows with guards.
- Make sure your child wears a bike helmet.
- Keep a vigilant eye on your little "tornado." Children this age can find trouble in the blink of an eye.

Kitchen Accidents
During these early years, your child will want to accompany you and "help" you with everything you do. In the kitchen, this can be dangerous. Your child may reach for hot items on the stove or table. He may trip you as you go about your work, causing spills and, possibly, serious burns. Or, he may try to imitate you by trying to turn on the stove, iron, or microwave.

Intervention
- Keep your child safely contained in a playpen, or secured in a high chair while you are in the kitchen.
- Keep older children busy with supervised projects.
- Maintain tap water temperature below 120°F to prevent scalding.

Away from Home
And while you are busy making your home safe for your child, don't overlook safety away from home.

Intervention
- Never let your child play in driveways, streets, or alleys.
- Be careful at homes you visit. Homes without young children may not be childproofed. Combine that with the fact that your child will be curious and want to explore the new environment, and you have a recipe for injury.
- Keep in mind that grocery stores pose another hazard to young children. Isles are often piled high with canned and boxed items a child can easily overturn. If you put your child in a shopping chart, always use the safety strap, and never leave your child in a shopping cart alone—even for a minute. There is an old saying: Children don't have accidents; parents do. Prevent childhood injury with proper intervention.

Nutrition

Good nutrition provides energy for a growing child and is important to ensure normal growth, development, and physical activity. When you grew up, nutrition was neatly divided into four categories: meats and poultry, dairy, breads and cereals, and fruits and vegetables. If every meal contained one item from each category, you were getting a well-balanced diet. Not anymore.

New United States Department of Agriculture (USDA) recommendations are based on a pyramid diagram, and ratios are no longer 1 to 1, but are based on building blocks for a solid foundation of healthy eating. The American Dietetic Association's Child Nutrition and Health Campaign recommends the following food guide for children:

Food Guide Pyramid for Children
Food amounts equal one serving

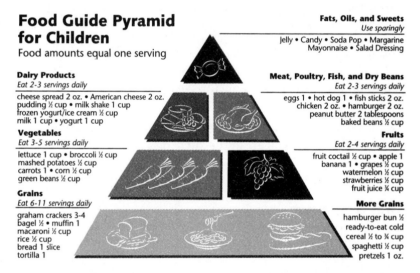

Fats, Oils, and Sweets
Use sparingly

Jelly • Candy • Soda Pop • Margarine
Mayonnaise • Salad Dressing

Dairy Products
Eat 2-3 servings daily

cheese spread 2 oz. • American cheese 2 oz.
pudding ½ cup • milk shake 1 cup
frozen yogurt/ice cream ½ cup
milk 1 cup • yogurt 1 cup

Meat, Poultry, Fish, and Dry Beans
Eat 2-3 servings daily

eggs 1 • hot dog 1 • fish sticks 2 oz.
chicken 2 oz. • hamburger 2 oz.
peanut butter 2 tablespoons
baked beans ½ cup

Vegetables
Eat 3-5 servings daily

lettuce 1 cup • broccoli ½ cup
mashed potatoes ½ cup
carrots 1 • corn ½ cup
green beans ½ cup

Fruits
Eat 2-4 servings daily

fruit coctail ½ cup • apple 1
banana 1 • grapes ½ cup
watermelon ½ cup
strawberries ½ cup
fruit juice ¾ cup

Grains
Eat 6-11 servings daily

graham crackers 3-4
bagel ½ • muffin 1
macaroni ½ cup
rice ½ cup
bread 1 slice
tortilla 1

More Grains

hamburger bun ½
ready-to-eat cold
cereal ½ to ¾ cup
spaghetti ½ cup
pretzels 1 oz.

In addition, make choosing, preparing, and eating food a pleasurable experience. Teach good habits that will last a lifetime. Research suggests that children who develop unhealthy eating patterns maintain those habits through adulthood, which can lead to increased risk of serious health problems.

To instill good nutrition habits in your children, practice the following suggestions:

- Make mealtimes pleasurable. Meals offer a time for the family to interact with one another. Eating together at the dinner table allows you to model good nutrition for your children.

- Give children healthy snacks, and convey the importance of limiting nonnutritious snacks. Teach children that nonnutritious snacks provide only empty calories; they do not provide nutrients to help the body grow. In addition, nonnutritious snacks, such as sweets, chips, and other junk foods, promote tooth decay and obesity.
- Resist the temptation to reward good behavior with sweets. In addition to the immediate damage (tooth decay and obesity), this practice encourages unhealthy attitudes toward food that can create lifelong problems.
- Set a good example with your eating and exercising habits. Children with obese parents are much more likely to have weight problems themselves, and the causes are probably environmental, not hereditary.
- If your child is overweight, most likely improper food choices and lack of exercise are responsible, not hormonal problems.

If your child exhibits consistently poor eating habits, or regularly skips meals, you may want to consult your physician about a nutrition screening and assessment. Once your child completes a questionnaire and undergoes a complete physical examination, your doctor can then determine your child's overall nutritional health and recommend appropriate nutrition education and counseling, if required.

Vitamins

Young children who generally eat a diet containing foods from the four food groups do not require vitamin supplementation.
- Breast-fed infants should receive 400 IUs of vitamin D daily, especially during winter months in cold climates where they may get very little sunlight.
- Iron-fortified formula is the ideal formula for bottle-fed babies during the first year. For breast-fed babies, iron-fortified formula should be used for the first year following weaning from the breast.
- Premature infants usually receive iron supplementation until the infant begins taking iron-containing food (cereals, meats, some vegetables) or has been switched to an iron-containing formula. Iron supplementation is not as usual for full-term infants.

Oral Health

Regular visits to your dentist are important to ensure optimal dental health. The American Academy of Pediatrics (AAP) and the American Association of Pediatric Dentistry have recently recommended earlier evaluation, between 12–18 months, or just after the primary teeth erupt. At these regular visits, your dentist will discuss oral hygiene (proper toothbrushing techniques, nutrition, the effects of pacifier use, thumbsucking, flossing, and so on).

The appropriate use of fluoride (drops and topical) is one of the most effective measures in preventing tooth decay. More than half the U.S. population resides in fluorinated-water areas; however, because of the quality of community water, many families use bottled water or have their own processing units, and so fluoride supplementaion is necessary. If you suspect your water is not properly fluorinated, ask your doctor about fluoride supplements and fluoride-testing laboratories.

However, dentists sometimes recommend fluoride supplements without conducting an appropriate water analysis. The excess fluoride may lead to fluorosis—a staining of the dental enamel.

PART TWO

Helping Your Child Get Better

Fever Guide

Fever Facts

- The body's "normal" temperature fluctuates between 97°F and 100.4°F, tending to be higher in the late afternoon.
- Rectal temperatures are approximately 1 degree higher than oral temperatures.
- Fever is not a disease; it is one of the body's defenses for fighting infection.
- High fevers do not necessarily indicate serious disease. Relatively harmless illnesses, such as roseola and other viral diseases, may cause high fevers. Also, some children tend to run high fevers with minor illnesses. Fever is considered high when it is above 104.5°F.
- High fevers do not injure the brain. Fever convulsions occur in less than 5 percent of children, and are generally harmless.
- The main reason for lowering a high temperature is to make your child feel more comfortable. Children generally experience little discomfort with temperatures below 102°F.

Taking Temperatures

Rectal temperatures are the most accurate and should be used for children under age 5. Armpit temperatures can be used if done correctly, but if the armpit temperature is elevated (above 101°F), it should be confirmed by a rectal temperature. Armpit temperature records the skin temperature and not the actual body temperature. To take an accurate armpit temperature, follow these instructions:

1. Place the tip of the thermometer in the armpit.
2. Hold the elbow against the chest for 4-5 minutes. (It is important to time this accurately.)
3. Confirm with a rectal temperature reading, if the armpit temperature is elevated.

Thermometers

- Thermometers other than standard glass and mercury models are available.
  —Digital thermometers are accurate and require less than 30 seconds to obtain a reading.
  —Ear thermometers' accuracy has been questioned, and they are relatively expensive.
  —Temperature strips are inaccurate.
- Do not use oral thermometers for children younger than age 5.

Treatment

- Do not use aspirin to treat a high temperature. Aspirin has been associated with a serious childhood condition called Reye's syndrome.
- Choose between the two drugs available for fever reduction: acetaminophen and ibuprofen. (Acetaminophen is available over the counter. Ibuprofen is available in some forms over the counter; other forms require a prescription. Acetaminophen and ibuprofen are equivalent in their fever-reduction potential. The advantage of ibuprofen is that it can be given every 6 hours and it helps reduce inflammation.)
- Do not alternate acetaminophen and ibuprofen every 2 hours in an attempt to improve fever control—this is not better than giving acetaminophen every 4 hours or ibuprofen every 6 hours, as recommended.
- Follow the dosages recommended by your health care professional or printed on the medication bottle.
- Make sure your child drinks plenty of fluids.
- Do not overdress children with fever.
- Sponge bathe your child only when necessary—generally only if the temperature remains over 104°F, 30–45 minutes after giving acetaminophen or ibuprofen. When a sponge bath is indicated, place your child in 2–3 inches of lukewarm water, and massage your child's body with a wet towel to prevent shivering.

When to Call Your Doctor about Fever

Call your doctor when

- an infant younger than 3–4 months has a rectal temperature over 100.4°F.
- children older than 3–4 months have a temperature of 103°F or higher. In most cases, your decision to call your doctor will be based on the associated symptoms (cough, sore throat, and so on).
- fever persists longer than 24 hours without other symptoms.

Acetaminophen Dosage Chart

Always read the label on any medication, ask your physician for dosage recommendations, and measure medicines accurately.

Age	Medication	Amount
Birth-3 Months (6–11 lbs.)	Infant's Drops[1]	½ dropperful
4–11 Months (12–17 lbs.)	Infant's Drops[1] Children's Liquid[2]	1 dropperful ½ tsp.
12–23 Months (18–23 lbs.)	Infant's Drops[1] or Children's Liquid[2]	1½ tsp. ¾ tsp.
2–3 Years (24–35 lbs.)	Infant's Drops[1] Children's Liquid[2] Children's Tablets[3]	2 tsp. 1 tsp. 2 tab.
4–5 Years (36–47 lbs.)	Children's Liquid[2] Children's Tablets[3]	1½ tsp. 3 tab.
6-8 Years (48–59 lbs.)	Children's Liquid[2] Children's Tablets[3] Junior Strength Tablets[4]	2 tsp. 4 tab. 2
9–10 Years (60–71 lbs.)	Children's Liquid[2] Children's Tablets[3] Junior Strength Tablets[4]	2½ tsp. 5 tab. 2½
11 Years (72–95 lbs.)	Children's Liquid[2] Children's Tablets[3] Junior Strength Tablets[4]	3 tsp. 6 tab. 3
12–14 Years (96 lbs. and over)	Junior Strength Tablets[4]	4

(Administer dozes 4-5 times daily, not to exceed 5 doses in 24 hours.)

[1]Infant's Suspension and Original Drops (80 mg/0.8 ml)
[2]Children's Suspension Liquid and Elixir (160 mg/5 ml):
[3]Children's Chewable Tablets (80 mg tabs)
[4]Junior Strength Chewable Tablets/Caplets (160 mg):

Ibuprofen Dosage Chart

Always read the label on any medication, ask your physician for dosage recommendations, and measure medicines accurately. (Note: Some forms of ibuprofen are available only by prescription.)

Age	P[1]/OTC[2]	Medication	Amount
6–11 Months	P	*Oral Drops (50 mg/1.25 ml)*	
(12–17 lbs.)		Fever under 102.5°F	½ dropperful
		Fever 102.5°F and over	1 dropperful
	P	*Suspension (100 mg/5 ml)*	
		Fever under 102.5°F	¼ tsp.
		Fever 102.5°F and over	½ tsp.
12–23 Months	P	*Oral Drops (50 mg/1.25 ml)*	
(18–23 lbs.)		Fever under 102.5°F	1 dropperful
		Fever 102.5°F and over	2 dropperfuls
	P	*Suspension (100 mg/5 ml)*	
		Fever under 102.5°F	½ tsp.
		Fever 102.5°F and over	1 tsp.
	P	*Chewable Tablets (50 mg)*	
		Fever under 102.5°F	1 tab
		Fever 102.5°F and over	2 tabs
	P	*Chewable Tablets (100 mg)*	
		Fever under 102.5°F	½ tab
		Fever 102.5°F and over	1 tab
2–3 Years	OTC	*Oral Drops (50 mg/1.25 ml)*	2 dropperfuls
(24–35 lbs.)	OTC	*Suspension (100 mg/5 ml)*	1 tsp.
	P	*Chewable Tablets (50 mg)*	
		Fever under 102.5°F	1½ tabs
		Fever 102.5°F and over	3 tabs
	P	*Chewable Tablets (100 mg)*	
		Fever under 102.5°F	¾ tab
		Fever 102.5°F and over	1½ tabs
4–5 Years	OTC	*Suspension (100 mg/5 ml)*	1½ tsp.
(36–47 lbs.)	P	*Chewable Tablets (50 mg)*	
		Fever under 102.5°F	2 tabs
		Fever 102.5°F and over	4 tabs
	P	*Chewable Tablets (100 mg)*	
		Fever under 102.5°F	1 tab
		Fever 102.5°F and over	2 tabs

Age	P[1]/OTC[2]	Medication	Amount
6–8 Years	OTC	*Suspension (100 mg/5 ml)*	2 tsp.
(48–59 lbs.)	P	*Chewable Tablets (50 mg)*	
		Fever under 102.5°F	2½ tabs
		Fever 102.5°F and over	5 tabs
	P	*Chewable Tablets (100 mg)*	
		Fever under 102.5°F	1¼ tabs
		Fever 102.5°F and over	2½ tabs
	OTC	*Caplets (100 mg)*	2 caps
9–10 Years	OTC	*Suspension (100 mg/5 ml)*	2½ tsp.
(60–71 lbs.)	P	*Chewable Tablets (50 mg)*	
		Fever under 102.5°F	3 tabs
		Fever 102.5°F and over	6 tabs
	P	*Chewable Tablets (100 mg)*	
		Fever under 102.5°F	1½ tabs
		Fever 102.5°F and over	3 tabs
	OTC	*Caplets (100 mg)*	2½ caps
11 Years	OTC	*Suspension (100 mg/5 ml)*	3 tsp.
(72–95 lbs.)	P	*Chewable Tablets (50 mg)*	
		Fever under 102.5°F	4 tabs
		Fever 102.5°F and over	8 tabs
	P	*Chewable Tablets (100 mg)*	
		Fever under 102.5°F	2 tabs
		Fever 102.5°F and over	4 tabs
	OTC	*Caplets (100 mg)*	3 caps

(Note: Dosages should be based on your child's weight, when possible.)
[1]Prescription
[2]Over-the-Counter

Is This an Emergency?

How do you determine whether your child's condition requires a trip to the emergency room? Certain warning signs always warrant a call to your doctor's office for advice. If you are able to reach your physician during office hours, you will be instructed whether to proceed to the office or the emergency room. If you think your child is seriously ill or has sustained a significant injury after office hours, call your doctor before you take your child directly to an emergency room or urgent care clinic. Your doctor may save you a visit.

Serious Warning Signs

Call your doctor immediately if your child exhibits any of the following serious symptoms:

- uncontrolled bleeding
- difficulty breathing or excessive drooling (with fever)
- cyanosis (blue color of the skin or lips)
- convulsions/seizures
- stupor or coma (unconsciousness)
- head injury with unconsciousness, confusion, or vomiting
- possibly serious accident or injury (especially neck injuries)
- fall from a significant height—even if serious injury is not obvious
- ingestion of a known or suspected poison
- major dental injury (such as a displaced tooth)
- obvious broken bone
- burns with blistering (secondary) or burns covering extensive areas of the body
- fever greater than 105°F
- blood in the urine, stool, or vomit
- severe pain that lasts longer than 5 minutes or recurs frequently
- swallowing or choking on a foreign object

What to Do in an Emergency

What you do in an emergency is just as important as getting your child the help she needs.

- First, stay calm. Call your local emergency number (911), or notify your doctor. Be ready with the following information: What happened? When? How old is your child? What symptoms is she exhibiting?
- If you are instructed to go to an emergency facility, know the quickest route. If you must contact an ambulance service yourself, tell the emergency medical technicians which hospital you prefer, if your child's condition and time permits.
- When you arrive at the emergency facility, make sure your doctor is notified. Your doctor can arrange specialized care for your child, should she require it.
- Post the following information near your phone. Update often.

EMERGENCY TELEPHONE NUMBER: _____

HOSPITAL NAME: _____

DOCTOR'S NAME AND TELEPHONE NUMBER: _____

First-Aid Supplies

The following supplies should be stocked in every home to treat both minor and serious injury until a doctor can be contacted. As with any medical supplies, these items should be stored out of children's reach.

- Adhesive bandages: assorted sizes
- Adhesive tape: ½ to 1 inch (1¼ to 2½ cm) wide
- Antibiotic ointment
- Antihistamines (over-the-counter)
- Antiseptic wipes or solution
- Band-Aids
- Calamine lotion
- Cool-mist vaporizer
- Cotton balls
- Cotton swabs
- Elastic bandages
- Heating pad or hot-water bottle
- Pain-relieving tablets or liquid (acetaminophen, ibuprofen)
- Scissors with blunt tips
- Sterile eyewash
- Sterile gauze bandages and pads
- Syrup of ipecac
- Thermometer (oral, ear, rectal, or digital)
- Triangular bandages and safety pins
- Tweezers (round-ended)

Treatments and Procedures

Compresses

Heating pads, hot water bottles, gauze, washcloths, towels, commercial (3M) ice packs, Popsicles, and ice cubes in plastic bags all can serve as compresses. Refer to specific entries in the treatment section to determine what kind of compress is best for a given injury or ailment.

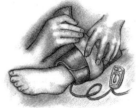
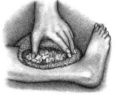

heating pad   cold compress

- Wet a towel or washcloth with hot or cold water; wring and fold. Or wrap an ice cube in a washcloth. Apply to face, back, joints, limbs, as necessary (put in plastic bag if moisture isn't necessary).
- Apply a plastic bag filled with ice (or a Popsicle) to mouth injuries.
- Press a wad of gauze or other clean cloth to a bleeding wound and hold firmly in place to reduce flow of blood.

Bandages

Adhesive bandages, gauze pads, tape, and elastic bandages help protect wounds from injury and promote healing.

- *Basic bandage:* Stop bleeding and clean wound before applying a gauze pad or adhesive bandage (tape if needed).
- *Elastic bandage:* Stop bleeding and apply dressings if needed, then wrap with even, gentle pressure. Unwrap several times a day if your doctor recommends it.
- *Butterfly closure* (for closing long or deep cuts): Cut ½-inch adhesive tape as shown; twist one end 360° until both ends have adhesive sides down. Push edges of wound together and apply; then cover with gauze or an adhesive bandage.

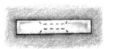
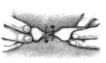

1. Cut as shown.   2. Twist 360°.   3. Push edges of wound together and apply.

- *Removing bandages:* Leave bandages in place 24 hours unless you're directed otherwise. Then remove and change bandages as necessary. Soak gauze in cold water before removing it; remove in direction of wound (rather than across it) to avoid disturbing the scab.

Splints

A splint is used to immobilize an injured body part and protect it from further injury. In general, do not try to move or reposition a fractured bone or dislocated joint. Always immobilize it in the position in which it was found. When splinting a body part, follow these general steps:

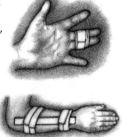

1. Use something rigid and flat for the splint, such as a board, ruler, stick, or rolled-up magazine or newspaper. You can also use a pillow or blanket, or, in some cases, another body part, such as a leg or finger.
2. Pad a hard or rigid splint with cloths or towels before attaching it.
3. Be certain the splint extends to the joints above and below a fracture.
4. Tie the splint to the injured body part with cloth strips, tape, belts, or neckties. Be careful not to attach the splint too tightly; if the fingers or toes become pale and cool, loosen the splint. Do not let knots press against the injured area.

Slings

A sling is used to immobilize an injured shoulder, collarbone, or forearm and place it in a comfortable position. Follow these general steps when making a sling:

1. Make a triangular sling by folding a square yard of cloth diagonally, or improvise by using an item of clothing.

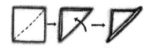

2. Have your child support his injured arm while you slip the sling under the arm, as shown.
3. Fold the cloth around the arm and pull the edges up over your child's shoulders.
4. Tie a knot on the side of your child's neck. Pin up the extra cloth at the elbow.
5. Tie the sling to your child's body with another piece of cloth, knotting the cloth on the uninjured side, to decrease mobility with some injuries.

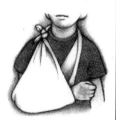

Bleeding Control

- Direct pressure will stop most bleeding. But if bleeding cannot be controlled or is associated with a serious injury, call your local emergency number (911). If bleeding continues, observe your child for shock. If your child becomes dizzy or faint and/or develops pale, cool, clammy skin, displays rapid, shallow breathing, and has a weak, rapid pulse, continue to treat the bleeding and see Shock, page 182.
- If you think a wound may need stitches, or if embedded gravel or dirt cannot be removed easily with gentle cleaning, take your child to an emergency facility. Prompt treatment is important to avoid secondary infection.
- Bleeding from the scalp is not always as serious as it seems; a small cut can appear to bleed profusely.

If your child is bleeding, follow these steps:

1. Calm and reassure your child.
2. Apply direct pressure to the wound with a clean, dry cloth. Maintain firm but gentle pressure for 5–10 minutes or until the bleeding subsides. If blood soaks through the cloth, do not remove it; you may loosen the clot. Place another cloth over the first one.
3. If the wound is superficial, wash it with soap and warm water and pat dry. Do not wash a wound that is deep or bleeding profusely. If you are unsure about the seriousness of the wound, call your doctor.
4. When the bleeding has subsided, even if the wound is still oozing, place a clean dressing over the wound. Bandage the dressing firmly, but not so tightly that the child's skin beyond the wound becomes pale and cool, which indicates that circulation is being cut off.

Caution: DO NOT apply a tourniquet to control bleeding; doing so may cause more harm than good.

Child Anatomy

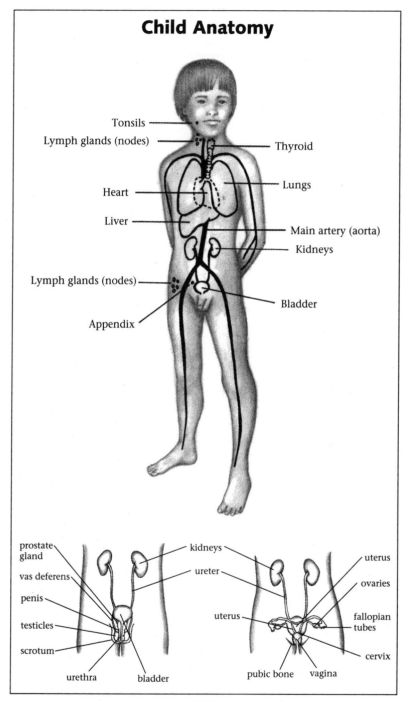

Tonsils

Lymph glands (nodes)

Thyroid

Heart

Lungs

Liver

Main artery (aorta)

Kidneys

Lymph glands (nodes)

Appendix

Bladder

prostate gland

kidneys

uterus

vas deferens

ureter

ovaries

penis

fallopian tubes

testicles

uterus

scrotum

cervix

urethra

bladder

pubic bone

vagina

PART THREE

Step-by-Step Treatments

When your child is ill or injured, you may have to react quickly. The recommendations in this section are not intended to replace professional guidance. Always address specific concerns to your health care professional. Frequently, there is more than one approach to medical problems; thus, your medical professional may have somewhat different recommendations than those in this book. Depending on the problem, your doctor may request an office visit or prescribe treatment over the telephone. Telephone instructions should always include specific guidelines as to when to call back or when to schedule an office visit if the child shows no improvement.

Remember, doctors are not infallible and cannot always make a specific diagnosis early in the course of an illness. Often, with time, the diagnosis becomes clear. A good example is the child who has fever for less than 8–12 hours without specific symptoms. Frequently, symptoms appear in the second 12 hours. When the symptoms develop, the doctor may then be able to clarify the diagnosis.

Description: A skin rash that usually occurs on the face and occasionally on the back and chest.

What you need to know:	When to get help:
• Acne should be treated aggressively. It may result in permanent scarring, and since adolescents are very self-conscious, acne may cause adverse emotional consequences. • It is not caused or worsened by chocolate, junk food, or lack of cleanliness. • Acne is probably caused by overproduction of sebum (material produced from fatty glands) and an increase in specific bacteria in the face.	• Call your doctor if your adolescent has a poor response to home treatment after 2–3 weeks.

Signs and symptoms:
• whiteheads (pimples with light centers)
• blackheads (pimples with dark centers)

Treatment:
• Wash with mild soap and water once or twice a day.
• Use makeup sparingly, and always remove cosmetics at night.
• Maintain a normal diet; there are no dietary restrictions.
• Apply 5% Benzyl Peroxide (over-the-counter) topically.
• Avoid "pimple popping," "blackhead popping," and excessive scrubbing.

Description: Facial rash that develops in 20–30 percent of newborns.

What you need to know:	When to get help:
• Acne may last a few months.	• Call your doctor for diagnosis only.
• It is probably caused by maternal hormones transferred to the baby.	
• Acne is unsightly, but it disappears on its own (self-limited).	

Signs and symptoms:
• pimples (small red bumps)

Treatment:
• Wash with mild soap and water.

Caution:
• Do not use oils or lotions that may block sweat glands and worsen the condition.

Description: Infection caused by the HIV virus resulting in a deterioration of the body's immune defense systems.

What you need to know:	**When to get help:**
• Most children acquire the virus before birth from HIV-positive mothers.	• Call your doctor if: —The signs or symptoms below are noted.
• AIDS is spread by sexual activity or from contact with HIV-infected blood.	—You have engaged in unsafe sexual practices with an unknown partner.
• Blood for transfusion is carefully screened for the HIV virus.	—You are injecting illegal drugs and are concerned about HIV.
• No child has developed the virus from normal play with other children.	

Signs and symptoms:
• frequent infections and fevers
• swollen glands
• chronic fatigue
• low birth weight or weight loss
• poor appetite
• chronic diarrhea

Treatment:
• Follow professional advice.
• For more information on AIDS and the HIV virus, call the National AIDS hotline at (800) 342-2437. Phone lines are open 7 days a week, 24 hours a day.

Description: An inherited physical reaction to one or more substances (pollen, dust, food, and so on).

What you need to know:	**When to get help:**
• Allergic symptoms do not occur on the first exposure to a substance; repeated exposure is required for sensitization. • Your child may be allergic if any of the below symptoms occur frequently or persist for extended periods. • Tobacco smoke worsens allergic respiratory symptoms.	• Call your doctor if your child develops hives or has difficulty breathing.

Signs and symptoms:
• watery eyes/runny nose
• itchy skin rash
• hives
• tingling lips and tongue
• itchy throat/swollen lips
• diarrhea
• nausea/vomiting
• dark circles under eyes
• difficulty breathing

Treatment:
• Follow the program prescribed by your doctor, which may include one or all of the following:
   —medications
   —dietary or environmental modification (for example, substituting cow's milk with soy milk, avoiding contact with wool, keeping the child's room free of dust)
   —allergy shots (less frequently)

Related topics: Asthma; Eczema; Hay Fever; Hives

Description: A shortage of hemoglobin (an oxygen-carrying substance) in the blood.

What you need to know:	**When to get help:**

• Anemia has many causes, including the following:
  —blood loss
  —accelerated breakdown of red blood cells
  —deficiency of iron in diet
  —insufficient production of red blood cells in the bone marrow
	• Call your doctor if you observe the below signs or symptoms, or you suspect your child is anemic.

Signs and symptoms:
- chronic fatigue, weakness
- paleness of fingernail beds and inside of eyelids
- shortness of breath
- rapid pulse
- jaundice

Treatment:
- Depends on the cause.
- Do not attempt home remedies.

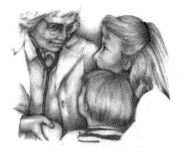

Related topics: Jaundice (in newborns); Leukemia

Description: A condition in which patients (usually middle-class adolescent females) suppress their urge to eat in order to lose weight.

What you need to know:	When to get help:
• Anorexia nervosa is a serious condition that requires constant supervision and specialized treatment.	• Call your doctor if you suspect anorexia nervosa, based on signs and symptoms.

Signs and symptoms:
• aversion to food
• excessive dieting
• excessive exercise
• self-induced vomiting
• distorted body image

Treatment:
• Follow the treatment program prescribed by your health care provider.

Description: An inflammation of the appendix that causes abdominal pain.

What you need to know:	When to get help:
• Sudden onset of severe pain in the abdomen is usually not appendicitis. • Children with appendicitis often lie still or walk with difficulty. • The appendix is attached to the large intestine and has no known function.	• Call your doctor if your child has localized pain, especially in the lower abdomen, lasting longer than 2–3 hours.

Signs and symptoms:
• constant pain that usually begins in the area of the navel and moves to the lower-right abdomen
• temperature of 101–102°F
• loss of appetite
• nausea/vomiting

Treatment:
• Apply a warm heating pad to the abdomen with onset of pain.
• Monitor your child's pain and temperature for 2–3 hours before consulting your physician.
• If appendicitis is suspected, surgery is indicated.

Caution:
• Do not give pain medications.
• Do not give laxatives if appendicitis is a possibility.

Related topics: "Stomach Pain" (Abdominal Pain)

Description: Inflammation of joints.

What you need to know:
- Arthritis may be an acute condition caused by infection and requires immediate treatment.
- There are many causes of arthritis. Lab tests may be necessary to make a specific diagnosis.

When to get help:
- Call your doctor if:
  —Your child's joints are red and swollen, especially if associated with fever.
  —The below signs and symptoms persist.

Signs and symptoms:
- joint swelling, aching, or tenderness
- difficulty moving joints without discomfort
- joint inflammation (redness)

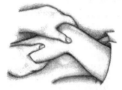

Treatment:
- Consult your doctor immediately if you suspect arthritis.
- Immobilize (rest) the joint involved.

Description: A reversible reaction in the air passages (bronchial tubes) caused by spasm inflammation of the lining and excessive mucus production.

What you need to know:	When to get help:
• All children who wheeze do not necessarily have asthma. There are other causes. • An asthma attack may have numerous triggers; most common are viruses, cold air, excessive exercise, and allergenic substances. • All asthma attacks require treatment.	• Call your doctor if your child's asthma attack is not relieved after taking prescribed medication.

Signs and symptoms:
- difficulty breathing, especially exhaling
- wheezing (high-pitched breathing sounds)
- coughing
- chest discomfort

Treatment:
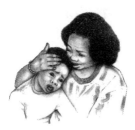

- Reassure your child; panic increases the severity of an asthma attack.
- Give prescribed medicines.
- Follow additional treatment measures as recommended by your doctor, which may include
  —environmental control,
  —shots (to increase resistance to certain allergens),
  —specific exercise programs.

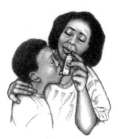

- Avoid irritants—tobacco, smoke, paint fumes, and so on.

Caution:
- Do not use over-the-counter nonprescription medications unless instructed by your physician.

Related topics: Allergy; Bronchiolitis; Bronchitis; Croup; Eczema; Hay Fever

Description: Infection of the skin of the foot, usually occuring between the toes, caused by a fungus.

What you need to know:	**When to get help:**
• Athlete's foot is rare in young children, common in adolescents. • The fungus associated with athlete's foot is acquired at pools, gyms, and showers.	• Call your doctor if home remedies do not relieve symptoms.

Signs and symptoms:
- itching
- redness
- cracking
- scaling
- blisters

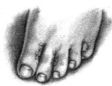

Treatment:
- Apply over-the-counter or prescribed antifungal ointment.
- Dry feet thoroughly after washing.
- Wear well-ventilated shoes.

Related topics: Ringworm

Description: Possible fracture of the back or neck, often caused by a blow or fall.

What you need to know:	When to get help:
• The signs and symptoms of a head or neck injury may occur immediately, or they may develop slowly over several hours.	• If the injury is to the back or neck, call your local emergency number (911) immediately.

Signs and symptoms:
- stiff neck
- pain in the neck area
- head held in unusual position
- weakness
- paralysis of extremities
- difficulty walking
- shock

Treatment:
Caution:

    —Do not bend, twist, or lift your child's head or body.

    —Do not try to move your child before medical help arrives.

    —Do not remove a helmet if your child is wearing one.

• If your child is unconscious, check for breathing.

• If your child isn't breathing, begin CPR.

• When your child resumes regular breathing, use rolled-up towels to immobilize your child's head and torso in the position found. (If emergency personnel are on the way, no further treatment is needed.)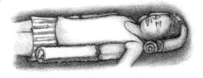

• If you *must* move your child, get several people to help. Keep the body as stable as possible.

Description: Pain or discomfort, usually secondary to muscle injury.

What you need to know:
- Most backaches result from muscle injury or overuse.
- Severe or localized pain may indicate a more serious problem.

When to get help:
- Call your doctor if:
  —The back pain is severe or localized.
  —Your child has fever greater than 101°F.
  —Pain extends to the legs.
  —Home treatment does not improve symptoms in 24–36 hours.

Signs and symptoms:
- localized pain, usually following specific movements

Treatment:
- Apply heat.
- Monitor temperature.
- Give acetaminophen or ibuprofen.
- Rest.
- Increase activity gradually.

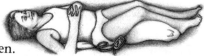

Description: Inability to control the bladder during sleep (after the child can be expected to do so).

What you need to know:	When to get help:
• Bedwetting is not deliberate.	• Call your doctor if:
• Most bedwetting resolves by age 6.	—Wetting occurs during the day, or during day and night.
• You should avoid punishing your child.	—Wetting recurs after the child has been dry for an extended period.
• Reducing fluids before bedtime or waking the child during the night is usually not effective.	—Wetting is accompanied by fever, painful urination, or blood in the urine.
• Specific treatment is not indicated before age 6.	—Bedwetting continues after age 5 or 6.

Signs and symptoms:
• consistent failure to remain dry at night

Treatment:
• Use a rubber pad to protect sheets.
• Use a bedwetting alarm.
• Reward dry nights with a star chart or star calendar.

Related topics: Diabetes Mellitus; Urinary Tract Infection

Description: A discoloration or raised area on the skin, present at birth.

What you need to know:	**When to get help:**
• Strawberry marks or lumps should only be treated in specific situations, i.e., when there is excessive bleeding or they interfere with vital structures (eye, ear). • Most birthmarks disappear in time.	• Call your doctor if: —A birthmark grows rapidly. —You observe excessive bleeding or signs of infection. —A birthmark is extensive and disfiguring.

Signs and symptoms:

Strawberry Mark (Hemangioma)

• flat or raised lump shaped like a strawberry (collection of small blood vessels)

• often not visible at birth and increases in size for weeks or months after

• gradually fades and disappears by age 5–6 years

• may require treatment if large enough to obstruct vital structures (eye, ear)

"Stork Bite" (Salmon Patch)

• flat, red, or salmon-colored marks on forehead, back, neck, or upper eyelid

• disappear in the first year

Mongolian Spot

• blue-black spots on lower back and buttocks

• look like bruises and eventually disappear

• most common in African American and Asian babies

Port Wine Stain

• red mark, often on forehead and face

• may require treatment if extensive, or disfiguring

Treatment:

• Laser treatment is often used when indicated.

Description: Bites by humans, pets, and animals, such as skunks, raccoons, and so on.

What you need to know:
- Puncture wounds—which are common with cat and human bites—pose the highest risk of infection. Dog bites are more superficial, and so have a lower incidence of infection.
- Rabies are a particular concern with bats, skunks (North American only), foxes, and stray cats and dogs. Observe the animal's behavior.
- Rabies are not a concern with squirrels, rabbits, hamsters, gerbils, and other rodents.

When to get help:
- Call your doctor if:
  —The bite broke the skin.
  —The bite looks infected.
  (Or, take your child to an emergency facility.)
- Call your local emergency number (911) if your child has multiple bites and/or severe bleeding.

Signs and symptoms:
- punctures (cat bites)
- crushed-looking wound (humans and dogs)

Treatment:
- If the bite is bleeding profusely, apply direct pressure with a clean, dry cloth until bleeding subsides.
- Wash the bite with soap and lukewarm running water for 3–5 minutes, and pat dry.
- Cover the bite with a clean dressing.
- Over the next 24–48 hours, observe the bite for signs of infection (increasing redness, swelling, pain).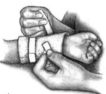
- Dog bites may occasionaly need stitches.
- Cat and human bites require antibiotic treatment, as determined by your doctor.

Caution:
- Do not clean the bite with alcohol or hydrogen peroxide, which may injure normal tissue.

Related topics: Breathing Emergency; Shock; Tetanus ("Lock Jaw")

Description: Bites by snakes, poisonous and nonpoisonous.

What you need to know:	When to get help:
• The bite of a poisonous snake is distinguished from a nonpoisonous snake bite by the presence of 1 or more fang marks on the skin.	• Call your local emergency number (911) if the bite is from a poisonous snake—or if you are uncertain whether the snake is poisonous. Or, immediately take your child to a hospital. Time is of the essence. If possible, call the hospital so antivenin can be ready when you arrive.

Signs and symptoms:
• one or two fang marks in the skin
• burning
• swelling
• pain
• discoloration
If venom enters the bloodstream:
• nausea
• vomiting
• shock (clammy skin; shallow breathing; weak, rapid pulse)

Treatment:
• Keep your child calm, restrict movement, and keep the affected area below heart level to reduce the flow of venom.
• Cover the bite with a clean, cool compress or a clean, moist dressing to reduce swelling and discomfort.

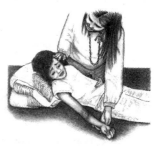

Caution:
• Do not give your child anything by mouth.
• Do not apply a tourniquet, make incisions in the wound, or suction the venom; doing so may cause more harm than good.

Related topics: Breathing Emergency; Shock; Tetanus ("Lock Jaw")

Description: Bites by insects.

What you need to know:	**When to get help:**
• Severe reactions to bee stings are very uncommon and usually—not always—occur shortly after the sting. • If your child experiences a severe reaction, additional evaluation by your doctor is indicated.	• Call your doctor if: —Your child has a rash. —The bite looks infected. (Or, take your child to an emergency facility.) • Call your local emergency number (911) if your child has difficulty breathing.

Signs and symptoms:

Mild Reaction
• pain
• redness
• 1–2 inches of swelling around the bite

Severe Reaction
• rash
• itching
• hives
• coughing
• wheezing
• difficulty breathing

Treatment:
• If the sting is from a honey bee, remove the stinger.
• Wash the site with soap and lukewarm water. If calamine lotion is available, dab some on the affected area to reduce discomfort.
• Cover the site with a clean, cold compress or a clean, moist dressing to reduce swelling and discomfort.
• Over the next 24–48 hours, observe the site for signs of infection (increasing redness, swelling, pain).

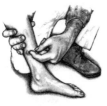
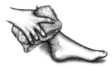

Related topics: Breathing Emergency; Shock; Tetanus ("Lock Jaw")

Description: A collection of fluid between layers of skin.

What you need to know:	**When to get help:**
• Blisters have multiple causes, which may include heat, burns, rubbing, chemical burns, infection (viruses or bacteria), or allergy.	• Call your doctor if: —Blisters look infected, or if redness or swelling extends outward. —Your child has multiple blisters.

Signs and symptoms:
• appearance of fluid under a raised layer of skin

Treatment:
• If the blister is intact, apply a gauze bandage.
• If the blister is broken, clean with soap and water, and apply antibiotic ointment.

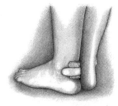

Caution:
• Do not pop "blisters"; they heal by themselves in a couple of days. Popping them may cause infection.

Related topics: Athlete's Foot; Burn; Chicken Pox; Cold Sore (Fever Blister); Hand, Foot, and Mouth Disease; Herpes Simplex Infection; Impetigo; Poison Ivy

Description: Infection in the bloodstream or lymph channels.

What you need to know:
- Infection from a wound often spreads initially through lymph channels to lymph nodes, which may contain the infection and prevent it from entering the bloodstream.
- Actual bloodstream infection is very serious and requires immediate evaluation and treatment. Antibiotics are usually required.

When to get help:
- Call your doctor immediately.
- Watch for
  —fever greater than 101°F
  —child acting ill
  —red streaks extending from wound
  —puss from lesion

Signs and symptoms:
- fever
- red streaks extending from wound, blister, or swollen gland (usually in lymph channels, not blood)

Treatment:
- There is no home treatment for blood poisoning.

Related topics: Boil; Cuts, Wounds, Scrapes

Description: A localized skin infection characterized by a painful collection of pus.

What you need to know:	When to get help:
• Boil is usually caused by staph bacteria.	• Call your doctor if:
• If pus drains from boil, it may spread to other parts of the body or to other people.	—Boils are multiple.
	—Fever is present.
	—Your child feels ill.
• If boil drains, dab with clean cloth or gauze pads.	—The boil does not drain in 2–3 days.
• Doctors frequently prescribe antibiotics.	

Signs and symptoms:
• painful red lump with whitish-yellow fluid

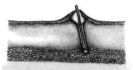

Treatment:
• Soak frequently—3–4 times a day, for 10–20 minutes—in Epsom salts or warm water until boil ruptures.
• Apply antibiotic ointment with warm compress after boil breaks.

Related topics: "Blood Poisoning"

Description: Legs bent outward, and knees farther apart than usual.

What you need to know:	When to get help:
• Most infants and children are bowlegged to some degree. • The condition is usually noted when child begins to walk. • Bowlegs usually correct spontaneously by age 3–4 years, and treatment is rarely indicated. • Bowlegs are rarely caused by a bone disorder or rickets. • Do not use special shoes unless recommended by your doctor.	• Call your doctor if the condition worsens over several months. • Ask your doctor about bowlegs at your child's routine health supervision examination.

Treatment:
• None, unless recommended by your doctor.

Description: Temporary enlargement of breasts in infants or adolescent males.

What you need to know:
- Hormone passage from mother to baby may cause breast enlargement in infants.
- Approximately 50–75 percent of boys develop some breast enlargement near puberty.
- Breast enlargement resolves without treatment in 1–2 years in adolescence and in 1 month in newborns.

When to get help:
- Call your doctor if:
  —Your adolescent is self-conscious or concerned about breast enlargement.
  —Your young infant develops pubic hair in addition to breast enlargement.

Signs and symptoms:
- mildly enlarged breast on one or both sides
- slight tenderness (especially in early adolescence)

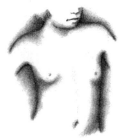

Treatment:
- None.

Description: Temporary stoppage of breathing often associated with excessive crying (temper tantrum) or an injury (such as a fall).

What you need to know:	**When to get help:**
• Breath-holding is not life threatening. • It is a type of temper outburst or tantrum. • Remain calm and treat breath-holding matter-of-factly. • Don't pour cold water on your child. • Breath-holding occurs most often between age 15 months and 3 years.	• Call your doctor if spells become habitual or occur frequently. • Call your local emergency number (911) if the spell lasts longer than 1 minute or the child is younger than age 6 months.

Signs and symptoms:
• red face initially, may become pale or blue
• occasionally jerking of the arms and legs (brief seizure)
• brief period of unconsciousness

Treatment:
• Be certain your child is in no danger of hurting herself if she falls.
• Do not be overly concerned.

Related topics: Convulsion

Description: A life-threatening situation resulting from a blocked airway, electric shock, or other condition.

What you need to know:	**When to get help:**
• The procedures for cardiopulmonary resuscitation (CPR) described below are not a substitute for CPR training. CPR training is necessary to perform these procedures safely and effectively. • If choking is the cause of breathing difficulty, follow the procedures for Choking, pages 76–79.	• If you are not alone, have one person call your local emergency number (911), while another person begins CPR. • If you are alone, shout HELP! If you are trained in CPR, administer CPR for about 1 minute, then call your local emergency number (911). • If you are alone and not trained in CPR, immediately call your local emergency number (911); emergency personnel will tell you what to do.

Treatment:

1 Rub your infant's back or tap his shoulder to determine whether he is conscious.

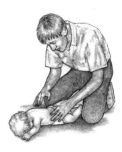

2 If the infant doesn't respond, turn him on his back onto a hard surface. Turn your infant as a unit, keeping his back in a straight line, firmly supporting his head and neck. Expose his chest.

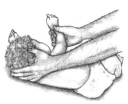

3 Lift your infant's chin while tilting his head back to move his tongue away from his windpipe. If you suspect a spinal injury, pull his jaw forward without moving his head or neck. Do not let his mouth close.

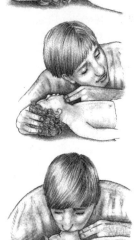

4 Place your ear close to your infant's mouth and watch for chest movement. For 5 seconds, look, listen, and feel for breathing.

5 If your infant is not breathing, begin rescue breathing as follows: Maintain his head position and cover his mouth and nose tightly with your mouth. Give 2 slow, gentle breaths, each lasting 1 to 1½ seconds. Pause between the 2 breaths so you can take a deep breath.

6 If you don't see your infant's chest rise, reposition his head and give 2 more breaths. If his chest still doesn't rise, his airway is obstructed; see Choking, pages 76–79.

7 If you do see your infant's chest rise, place two fingers on the inside of his upper arm, just above the elbow. Squeeze gently to feel his pulse for 5–10 seconds.

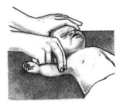

8 If your infant has a pulse, give 1 breath every 3 seconds. Check his pulse after every 20 breaths (each minute). After 1 minute, call your local emergency number (911). Resume giving breaths and checking the pulse.

9 If your infant has no pulse, begin chest compressions, as follows: Maintain his head position and place 2 fingers on the middle of his breastbone, just below his nipples. Within 3 seconds, quickly press your fingers down ⅓ to ½ inch the depth of his chest 5 times. Give the compressions in a smooth, rhythmic manner, keeping your fingers on his chest.

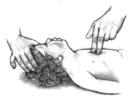

10 Give your infant 1 breath, followed by 5 chest compressions. Repeat this sequence 10 times.

11 Recheck your infant's pulse for 5–10 seconds.

12 Repeat steps 10 and 11 until your infant's pulse resumes or help arrives. If your infant's pulse resumes, go to Step 8.

Caution:
• Do not give chest compressions if there is a heartbeat; doing so may cause the heart to stop beating.
• If you suspect a spinal injury, do not move your infant's head or neck to check for breathing.

Description: A life-threatening situation resulting from a blocked airway, electric shock, or other condition.

What you need to know:	When to get help:
• The procedures for cardiopulmonary resuscitation (CPR) described below are not a substitute for CPR training. CPR training is necessary to perform these procedures safely and effectively. • If choking is the cause of breathing difficulty, follow the procedures for Choking, pages 80–83.	• If you are not alone, have one person call your local emergency number (911), while another person begins CPR. • If you are alone, shout HELP! If you are trained in CPR, administer CPR for about 1 minute, then call your local emergency number (911). • If you are alone and not trained in CPR, immediately call your local emergency number (911); emergency personnel will tell you what to do.

Treatment:

1 Tap or shake your child gently and call her name to determine consciousness.

2 If the infant doesn't respond, turn her on her back onto a hard surface. Turn your child as a unit, keeping her back in a straight line, firmly supporting her head and neck. Expose her chest.

3 Lift your child's chin while tilting her head back to move her tongue away from her windpipe. If you suspect a spinal injury, pull your child's jaw forward without moving her head or neck. Do not let her mouth close.

4 Place your ear close to your child's mouth and watch for chest movement. For 5 seconds, look, listen, and feel for breathing.

5 If your child is not breathing, begin rescue breathing, as follows: Maintain her head position, close her nostrils by pinching them with your thumb and index finger, and cover her mouth tightly with your mouth. Give 2 slow, full breaths. Pause between the 2 breaths so you can take a deep breath.

6 If you don't see your child's chest rise, reposition her head and give 2 more breaths. If her chest still doesn't rise, her airway is obstructed; see Choking, pages 80–83.

7 If you do see your child's chest rise, place 2 fingers on her Adam's apple. Slide your fingers into the groove between the Adam's apple and the muscle on the side of her neck to feel her pulse for 5–10 seconds.

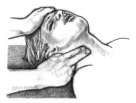

8 If your child has a pulse, give 1 breath every 4 seconds. Check her pulse after every 15 breaths. After 1 minute, call your local emergency number (911). Resume giving breaths and checking the pulse.

9 If your child has no pulse, begin chest compressions as follows: Maintain her head position and place the heel of your hand 2 finger-widths above the lowest notch of her breastbone. Lean your shoulders over your hand and within 4 seconds, quickly press down ⅓ to ½ inch the depth of her chest 5 times. Give the compressions in a smooth, rhythmic manner, keeping your hand on her chest.

10 Give your child 1 breath, followed by 5 chest compressions. Repeat this sequence 10 times.

11 Recheck her pulse for 5–10 seconds.

12 Repeat Steps 10 and 11 until your child's pulse resumes or help arrives. If her pulse resumes, go to Step 8.

Caution:
• Do not give chest compressions if there is a heartbeat; doing so may cause the heart to stop beating.
• If you suspect a spinal injury, do not move your child's head or neck to check for breathing.

Description: A life-threatening situation resulting from a blocked airway, electric shock, or other condition.

What you need to know:	When to get help:
• The procedures for cardiopulmonary resuscitation (CPR) described below are not a substitute for CPR training. CPR training is necessary to perform these procedures safely and effectively. • If choking is the cause of breathing difficulty, follow the procedures for Choking, pages 80–83.	• If you are not alone, have one person call your local emergency number (911), while another person begins CPR. • If you are alone, shout HELP! If you are trained in CPR, administer CPR for about 1 minute, then call your local emergency number (911). • If you are alone and not trained in CPR, immediately call your local emergency number (911); emergency personnel will tell you what to do.

Treatment:

1 Tap or shake your child gently, and call his name to determine consciousness.

2 If your child doesn't respond, turn him on his back onto a hard surface. Turn your child as a unit, keeping his back in a straight line, firmly supporting his head and neck. Expose his chest.

3 Lift your child's chin while tilting his head back to move his tongue away from his windpipe. If you suspect a spinal injury, pull your child's jaw forward without moving his head or neck. Do not let his mouth close.

4 Place your ear close to your child's mouth and watch for chest movement. For 5 seconds, look, listen, and feel for breathing.

5 If your child is not breathing, begin rescue breathing, as follows: Maintain his head position, close his nostrils by pinching them with your thumb and index finger, and cover his mouth tightly with your mouth. Give 2 slow, full breaths. Pause between the 2 breaths so you can take a deep breath.

6 If you don't see your child's chest rise, reposition his head and give 2 more breaths. If his chest still doesn't rise, his airway is obstructed; see Choking, pages 80–83.

7 If you do see your child's chest rise, place 2 fingers on his Adam's apple. Slide your fingers into the groove between the Adam's apple and the muscle on the side of his neck to feel his pulse for 5–10 seconds.

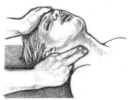

8 If your child has a pulse, give 1 breath every 5 seconds. Check his pulse after every 12 breaths. After 1 minute, call your local emergency number (911). Resume the breaths and pulse checks.

9 If your child has no pulse, begin chest compressions, as follows: Maintain his head position and place the heel of your hand 2 finger-widths above the lowest notch of his breastbone. Place the heel of your other hand directly over the heel of the first hand. Interlock your fingers; do not let them touch your child's chest. Lean your shoulders over your hands, and within 10 seconds quickly press down ⅓ to ½ inch the depth of his chest 15 times. Give the compressions in a smooth, rhythmic manner, keeping your hands on his chest.

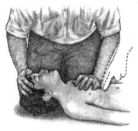

10 Give your child 2 breaths, followed by 15 chest compressions. Repeat this sequence 4 times. Recheck his pulse for 5–10 seconds.

11 Repeat Step 10 until your child's pulse resumes or help arrives. If his pulse resumes, go to Step 8.

Caution:
• Do not give chest compressions if there is a heartbeat; doing so may cause the heart to stop beating.
• If you suspect a spinal injury, do not move your child's head or neck to check for breathing.

Description: A crack or break in a bone that causes pain, swelling, bruising, deformity, limitation of movement, or pain on weight bearing.

What you need to know:	**When to get help:**
• A fracture is the cracking, breaking, or buckling of bones; a dislocation is the displacement or slippage of bones from joints. • Always immobilize a fractured or dislocated part in the position in which it was found.	• Call your doctor if your child has a fracture or dislocation; or take the child to an emergency facility.

Treatment:

1 Treat any bleeding with direct pressure. (See Treatments and Procedures: Bleeding Control, page 26.)

2 If the injury is to the shoulder or upper arm, immobilize the arm with a triangular cloth sling and tie the sling to the body. (See Treatments and Procedures: Slings, page 25 .)

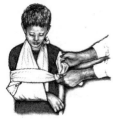

3 If the injury is to a limb or finger, immobilize the injured part—in the position in which it was found—with a padded splint. (See Treatments and Procedures: Splints, page 25.)

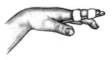

4 If the injury is to a forearm, after splinting it, place the arm in a triangular cloth sling and tie the sling to the body. (See Treatments and Procedures: Slings, page 25.)

5 If the injury is to the hip, pelvis, or thigh, and you are waiting for an ambulance, immobilize the injured area by placing rolled-up towels, blankets, or clothing between your child's legs. Do not let your child move her legs.

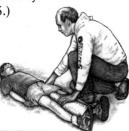

6 If the injury is to the hip, pelvis, or thigh, and you must move your child yourself, immobilize the injured body part on a stretcher. If possible, get several people to help. Use a sturdy board, such as an ironing board or another long, flat object that extends from the child's head to her heels. Together, roll her entire body as a unit—keeping the head, neck, and back in a straight line—toward you.

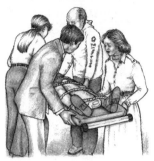

Slide the board alongside her. Roll her onto the board, again keeping the head and torso stable. Place rolled-up towels, blankets, or clothing between her legs. Use ropes, belts, tape, or strips of cloth to help hold her in place on the stretcher. Keep her as horizontal as possible when transporting her.

7 If your child is uncomfortable, apply cold compresses to the injury to reduce pain and swelling.

Caution:

• Call your local emergency number (911) if you suspect an injury to the spine, a severe head injury, multiple fractures, or if a chest injury is associated with difficulty breathing.

• If you suspect a spinal injury or a broken hip, pelvis, or thigh, do not move your child unless absolutely necessary. If you must move her, follow the directions above.

• Do not try to move or reposition a fractured or dislocated part.

Description: Inflammation and spasm causing narrowing of the small air passages (bronchioles) caused by viruses.

What you need to know:
• Bronchiolitis occurs in young children (under 2 years).
• It does not require antibiotic treatment.
• It is most often caused by the respiratory syncytial virus (RSV).

When to get help:
• Call your doctor if:
—Your child has difficulty breathing.
—Your child refuses fluids over 12–18 hours.

Signs and symptoms:
• rapid, labored breathing
• coughing
• wheezing
• fever (low grade, 101–102°F)

Treatment:
• Offer clear liquids.
• Administer oral and/or any inhaled medicine (if your doctor prescribes a special machine for administration of medicine) to open air passages.

Related topics: Asthma; Bronchitis; Pneumonia

Description: Inflammation of the air passages (bronchial tubes).

What you need to know:	**When to get help:**
• Bronchitis is often preceded by a cold.	• Call your doctor if:
• It is usually caused by viruses (in children) and does not require antibiotics.	—Your child has a temperature greater than 102.5°F.
• This diagnosis is rarely made in children.	—Your child refuses fluids over 12–18 hours.

Signs and symptoms:
• rapid breathing, sometimes labored
• wheezing
• coughing
• fever (usually low-grade)
• cold symptoms

Treatment:
• Increase fluids (helps moisten secretions).
• Administer medications prescribed by physician.

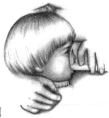

Related topics: Asthma; Bronchiolitis; Cold

Description: Discolored skin, sometimes swollen, indicating broken small blood vessels.

What you need to know:	When to get help:
• Bruises are usually secondary to an injury. • They may take weeks to disappear completely.	• Call your doctor if: —Bruises develop without a history of injury. —Bruises develop in association with fever or other signs of illness. —Broken bone symptoms (swelling, deformity, or pain on movement) are present.

Signs and symptoms:
• color may change from black to purple to yellow-brown

Treatment:
• Most bruises require no treatment.
• Apply cold pack to reduce bleeding and swelling (10 minutes on, 10 minutes off).

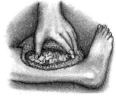

• After 24 hours, heat may speed disappearance of a bruise.

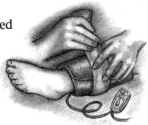

Description: An injury resulting from heat, hot liquids, electrical shock, chemicals, or radiation.

What you need to know:	When to get help:
• Burns that cover more than 10 percent of the body may require hospitalization.	• Go to an emergency facility for any chemical or electrical burn, or if you are uncertain about a burn's severity.

Signs and symptoms:

First-Degree Burns
(affect outer layer of skin)
• pain
• redness
• swelling

Second-Degree Burns
(affect both the outer and underlying layer of skin)
• pain
• redness
• swelling
• blistering

Third-Degree Burns
(extend into deeper skin tissues)
• may cause brown or blackened skin
• may be painless

Treatment:

1 If your child has a ***chemical burn,*** immediately remove all burned clothing and immerse the burned area in cool water under a tap or hose—or, if burns are extensive, place your child in a shower or bathtub—for 10 minutes. Pat dry. Go to Step 4.

2 If your child is ***on fire,*** either (a) douse him with water if it is available; (b) wrap him in thick, nonsynthetic material, such as a wool or cotton coat, rug, or blanket, to smother the flames; or (c) lay him flat and roll him on the ground. If your clothes catch fire, STOP, DROP, AND ROLL. When the fire is out, go to Step 3.

3 If your child has a ***heat, fire, or electrical burn***, remove any clothing that comes off easily and rinse the burned area in cool water under a shower, tap, or hose, depending on the

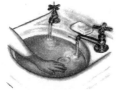

extent of the burn, until the pain subsides. Cover burned areas that cannot be immersed, such as the face, with wet cloths. Pat dry.

4 Cover the burned area with a clean, dry, nonfluffy dressing. If the burn is on your child's hands or feet, keep his fingers or toes apart by placing cloth or gauze between them; then loosely wrap the hand or foot in a clean dressing.

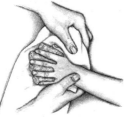

5 If the burn is **minor,** over the next 24–48 hours observe the area for signs of infection (increasing redness, swelling, and pain). If the burn looks infected, call your doctor or take your child to an emergency facility.

6 If the burn is extensive, and your child is not vomiting, give him liquids to help replace lost fluids.

Caution:
• Do not remove dead skin or break blisters.
• Do not apply ice, butter, ointments, medications, fluffy cotton dressings, or adhesive bandages to a burn.
• Call your local emergency number (911) if you have any concerns about a burn.

Related topics: Blister; Electric Shock; Sunburn

Description: Sores that develop on the inside of the mouth or on the lips.

What you need to know:	**When to get help:**
• Canker sores are not caused by viruses (herpes). • They are not contagious. • Sores may be recurrent. • They may last a week.	• Call your doctor if: —Multiple sores prevent your child from drinking or eating. —Same sores develop in other areas (gums, tongue, eyes).

Signs and symptoms:
• lesions inside mouth or on lips

Treatment:
• Apply antacid/antihistamine solution (sometimes prescribed by physician).
• Offer Popsicles.
• Give acetaminophen.

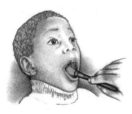

Related topics: Cold Sore (Fever Blister); Hand, Foot, and Mouth Disease; Herpes Simplex Infection

Description: A life-threatening condition when the heart stops beating.

What you need to know:	When to get help:
• The procedures for cardiopulmonary resuscitation (CPR) described below are not a substitute for CPR training. CPR training is necessary to perform these procedures most effectively and safely. • If choking is the cause of breathing difficulty, follow the procedures for Choking, pages 76–79 .	• If you are not alone, immediately have one person call your local emergency number (911), while another person begins CPR. • If you are alone, shout HELP! If you are trained in CPR, administer CPR for about 1 minute, then call your local emergency number (911). • If you are alone and not trained in CPR, immediately call your local emergency number (911); emergency personnel will tell you what to do.

Treatment:

1 Rub your infant's back or tap her shoulder to determine whether she is conscious.

2 If the infant doesn't respond, turn her on her back onto a hard surface. Turn your infant as a unit, keeping her back in a straight line, firmly supporting her head and neck. Expose her chest.

3 Lift your infant's chin while tilting her head back to move her tongue away from her windpipe. If you suspect a spinal injury, pull your infant's jaw forward without moving her head or neck. Do not let her mouth close.

4 Place your ear close to your infant's mouth and watch for chest movement. For 5 seconds, look, listen, and feel for breathing.

5 If your infant is not breathing, begin rescue breathing as follows: Maintain her head position and cover her mouth and nose tightly with your mouth. Give 2 slow, gentle breaths, each lasting 1 to 1½ seconds. Pause between the 2 breaths to take a deep breath.

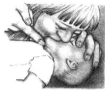

6 If you don't see your infant's chest rise, reposition her head and give 2 more breaths. If her chest still doesn't rise, her airway is obstructed; see Choking, pages 76–79.

7 If you do see your infant's chest rise, place two fingers on the inside of her upper arm, just above the elbow. Squeeze gently to feel her pulse for 5–10 seconds.

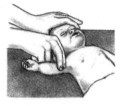

8 If your infant has a pulse, give 1 breath every 3 seconds. Check her pulse after every 20 breaths (each minute). After 1 minute, call your local emergency number (911). Resume giving breaths and checking the pulse.

9 If your infant has no pulse, begin chest compressions, as follows: Maintain her head position and place 2 fingers on the middle of her breastbone, just below her nipples. Within 3 seconds, quickly press your fingers down ⅓ to ½ inch the depth of her chest 5 times. Give the compressions in a smooth, rhythmic manner, keeping your fingers on her chest.

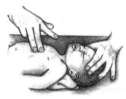

10 Give your infant 1 breath, followed by 5 chest compressions. Repeat this sequence 10 times. Recheck your infant's pulse for 5–10 seconds.

11 Repeat steps 10 until your infant's pulse resumes or help arrives. If your infant's pulse resumes, go to Step 8.

Caution:
• Do not give chest compressions if there is a heartbeat; doing so may cause the heart to stop beating.
• If you suspect a spinal injury, do not move your infant's head or neck to check for breathing.

Description: A life-threatening condition when the heart stops due to breathing emergency or other situation.

What you need to know:	When to get help:
• The procedures for cardiopulmonary resuscitation (CPR) described below are not a substitute for CPR training. CPR training is necessary to perform these procedures most effectively and safely. • If choking is the cause of breathing difficulty, follow the procedures for Choking, pages 80–83.	• If you are not alone, have one person call your local emergency number (911), while another person begins CPR. • If you are alone, shout HELP! If you are trained in CPR, administer CPR for about 1 minute, then call your local emergency number (911). • If you are alone and not trained in CPR, immediately call your local emergency number (911); emergency personnel will tell you what to do.

Treatment:

1 Tap or shake your child gently and call his name to determine consciousness.

2 If your child doesn't respond, turn him on his back onto a hard surface. Turn your child as a unit, keeping his back in a straight line, firmly supporting his head and neck. Expose his chest.

3 Lift your child's chin while tilting his head back to move his tongue away from his windpipe. If you suspect a spinal injury, pull your child's jaw forward without moving his head or neck. Do not let his mouth close.

4 Place your ear close to your child's mouth and watch for chest movement. For 5 seconds, look, listen, and feel for breathing.

5 If your child is not breathing, begin rescue breathing, as follows: Maintain his head position, close his nostrils by pinching them with your thumb and index finger, and cover his mouth tightly with your mouth. Give 2 slow, full breaths. Pause between the 2 breaths to take a deep breath.

6 If you don't see your child's chest rise, reposition his head and give 2 more breaths. If his chest still doesn't rise, his airway is obstructed; see Choking, pages 80–83.

7 If you do see your child's chest rise, place 2 fingers on his Adam's apple. Slide your fingers into the groove between the Adam's apple and the muscle on the side of his neck to feel his pulse for 5–10 seconds.

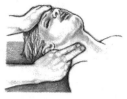

8 If your child has a pulse, give 1 breath every 4 seconds. Check his pulse after every 15 breaths. After 1 minute, call your local emergency number (911). Resume giving breaths and checking the pulse.

9 If your child has no pulse, begin chest compressions as follows: Maintain his head position and place the heel of your hand 2 finger-widths above the lowest notch of his breastbone. Lean your shoulders over your hand and within 4 seconds, quickly press down ⅓ to ½ inch the depth of his chest 5 times. Give the compressions in a smooth, rhythmic manner, keeping your hand on his chest.

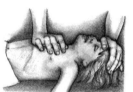

10 Give your child 1 breath, followed by 5 chest compressions. Repeat this sequence 10 times. Recheck his pulse for 5–10 seconds.

11 Repeat Step 10 until your child's pulse resumes or help arrives. If pulse resumes, go to Step 8.

Caution:
• Do not give chest compressions if there is a heartbeat; doing so may cause the heart to stop beating.
• If you suspect a spinal injury, don't move your child's head or neck to check for breathing.

Description: A life-threatening condition when the heart stops due to breathing emergency or other situation.

What you need to know:

- The procedures for cardiopulmonary resuscitation (CPR) described below are not a substitute for CPR training. CPR training is necessary to perform these procedures most effectively and safely.
- If choking is the cause of breathing difficulty, follow the procedures for Choking, pages 80–83.

When to get help:

- If you are not alone, have one person call your local emergency number (911), while another person begins CPR.
- If you are alone, shout HELP! If you are trained in CPR, administer CPR for about 1 minute, then call your local emergency number (911).
- If you are alone and not trained in CPR, immediately call your local emergency number (911); emergency personnel will tell you what to do.

Treatment:

1 Tap or shake your child gently, and call her name to determine consciousness.

2 If your child doesn't respond, turn her on her back onto a hard surface. Turn your child as a unit, keeping her back in a straight line, firmly supporting her head and neck. Expose her chest.

3 Lift your child's chin while tilting her head back to move her tongue away from her windpipe. If you suspect a spinal injury, pull your child's jaw forward without moving her head or neck. Do not let her mouth close.

4 Place your ear close to your child's mouth and watch for chest movement. For 5 seconds, look, listen, and feel for breathing.

5 If your child is not breathing, begin rescue breathing, as follows: Maintain her head position, close her nostrils by pinching them with your thumb and index finger, and cover her mouth tightly with your mouth. Give 2 slow, full breaths. Pause between the 2 breaths to take a deep breath.

6 If you don't see your child's chest rise, reposition her head and give 2 more breaths. If her chest still doesn't rise, her airway is obstructed; see Choking, pages 80–83.

7 If you do see your child's chest rise, place 2 fingers on her Adam's apple. Slide your fingers into the groove between the Adam's apple and the muscle on the side of her neck to feel her pulse for 5–10 seconds.

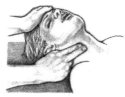

8 If your child has a pulse, give 1 breath every 5 seconds. Check her pulse after every 12 breaths. After 1 minute, call your local emergency number (911). Resume the breaths and pulse checks.

9 If your child has no pulse, begin chest compressions, as follows: Maintain her head position and place the heel of your hand 2 finger-widths above the lowest notch of her breastbone. Place the heel of your other hand directly over the heel of the first hand. Interlock your fingers; don't let them touch your child's chest. Lean your shoulders over your hands, and within 10 seconds quickly press down ⅓ to ½ inch the depth of her chest 15 times. Give the compressions in a smooth, rhythmic manner, keeping your hands on her chest.

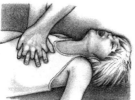

10 Give your child 2 breaths, followed by 15 chest compressions. Repeat this sequence 4 times. Recheck her pulse for 5–10 seconds.

11 Repeat Step 10 until your child's pulse resumes or help arrives. If her pulse resumes, go to Step 8.

Caution:
• Do not give chest compressions if there is a heartbeat; doing so may cause the heart to stop beating.
• If you suspect a spinal injury, don't move your child's head or neck to check for breathing.

Description: Illness caused by a bacteria from the scratch of a young cat (usually a kitten).

What you need to know:	When to get help:
• Kittens that scratch are not ill. • Most children improve without treatment.	• Call your doctor if: —Your child's glands become large, red, or tender. —Your child has received a cat bite, not only a scratch.

Signs and symptoms:
• fever
• large, tender, red lymph glands (neck, armpit)
• bumpy rash at or near site of scratch is an early sign
• cat scratch history

Treatment:
• Wash site of cat scratch thoroughly.
• Antibiotics may be prescribed by your physician in some cases.

Description: Highly contagious virus that causes an itchy rash with blisters.

What you need to know:
- One episode of chicken pox usually makes the child immune to this disease.
- The disease is contagious from one day before the rash appears until all the sores dry or crust.
- Do not give aspirin (it places child at risk of developing Reye's syndrome).
- Vaccine is now available that can be given between ages 12–18 months.

When to get help:
- Call your doctor if:
  —Your child's rash becomes infected (increasing redness or pus).
  —High fever, vomiting, disorientation, or convulsions occur.
  —Fever over 101°F persists beyond the fourth day— may be a sign of secondary strep infection.

Signs and symptoms:
- headache
- fatigue
- fever
- rash that progresses from red spots to blisters, which dry and form scabs
- itchy rash that appears in crops over several days, so is present in different stages simultaneously

Treatment:
- Give acetaminophen.
- Provide oatmeal or corn starch baths.
- Apply calamine lotion.
- Discourage scratching. Cut your child's fingernails or have her wear gloves to reduce damage from scratching.
- Administer medicine if prescribed by your physician.

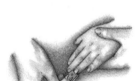

Related topics: Blister; Reye's Syndrome; Shingles

Description: A life-threatening obstruction of the airway by an object, food, or croup.

What you need to know:	**When to get help:**
• If breathing has stopped, DO NOT begin emergency breathing until the airway is cleared.	• If someone is with you, call your local emergency number (911), while the other person follows the first-aid steps. • If you are alone, shout HELP! If you can do so quickly, call your local emergency number (911). Then follow the first-aid steps below. • Call your doctor for further instructions, even if you dislodge the obstruction and your child seems fine.

Signs and symptoms:
• inability to breathe, cry, or make sounds
• high-pitched noises
• ineffective coughs
• bluish lips, nails, and skin

Treatment:

1 Lay your infant's face down along your forearm, with his chest in your hand and his jaw between your thumb and index finger. Use your thigh or lap for support. Keep your child's head lower than his body, turning his head to one side.

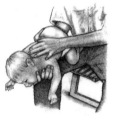

2 Give 5 quick, forceful blows, one per second, between your infant's shoulder blades with the heel of your other hand.

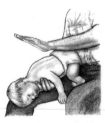

3 Turn your infant over so he is face up on your other arm. Use your thigh or lap for support. Keep his head lower than his body.

4 Place 2 fingers on the lower half of your infant's breastbone, one finger's breadth below his nipples.

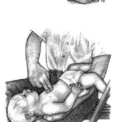

5 Thrust your fingers down quickly ⅓ to ½ inch the depth of his chest 5 times, at the rate of one per second.

6 If the object does not come out, turn your infant over so he is face down on your other arm and give another 5 back blows. Continue alternating 5 back blows with 5 chest thrusts until the object is dislodged, help arrives, or your infant loses consciousness. If your infant loses consciousness, read the next section: Choking— For Unconscious Infant Under 1 Year.

Caution:
• Do not interfere with your infant if he can still cough, breathe, or cry.
• Do not try to dislodge and remove the object if you cannot see it.
• Do not initiate first-aid steps until you are certain your infant is actually choking. If he can't cough or cry, or if his coughing and crying are very weak, then follow the first-aid steps above.

Description: A life-threatening obstruction of the airway by an object, food, or croup.

What you need to know:	When to get help:
• If breathing has stopped, DO NOT begin emergency breathing until the airway is cleared.	• If someone is with you, call your local emergency number (911), while the other person follows the first-aid steps. • If you are alone, shout HELP! If you can do so quickly, call your local emergency number (911). Then follow the first-aid steps below. • Call your doctor for further instructions, even if you dislodge the obstruction and your child seems fine.

Signs and symptoms:
• inability to breathe, cry, or make sounds
• high-pitched noises
• ineffective coughs
• bluish lips, nails, and skin

Treatment:

1 Firmly supporting your infant's head and neck, place her on her back onto a hard surface. Move your infant as a unit, keeping her back in a straight line. Expose her chest.

2 Open your infant's mouth with your thumb and index finger, placing your thumb over her tongue. *If the object is visible and loose, remove it with a hooked index finger.*

3 Look, listen, and feel for breathing. Lift your infant's chin while tilting her head back to move her tongue away from her windpipe. Do not let her mouth close. Place your ear close to her mouth and watch for chest movement. For 5 seconds, look, listen, and feel for breathing.

4 If your infant is not breathing, begin rescue breathing: Maintain her head position and cover her mouth and nose tightly with your mouth. Give 2 slow, gentle breaths, each lasting 1 to 1½ seconds. Pause between the 2 breaths to take a deep breath.

5 If you don't see your infant's chest rise, reposition her head and give 2 more breaths.

6 If your infant's chest still doesn't rise, begin back blows. Lay her face down along your forearm with her chest in your hand and her jaw between your thumb and index finger. Use your thigh or lap for support. Keep your child's head lower than her body, turning her head to one side.

7 Give 5 quick, forceful blows, 1 per second, between her shoulder blades with the heel of your other hand.

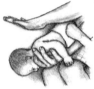

8 Turn your infant over so she is face up on your other arm. Use your thigh or lap for support. Keep her head lower than her body.

9 Place 2 fingers on the lower half of your infant's breastbone, one finger's breadth below her nipples.

10 Quickly thrust your fingers down ⅓ to ½ inch the depth of her chest 5 times, at the rate of 1 per second.

11 Open your infant's mouth with your thumb and index finger, placing your thumb over her tongue. *If the object is visible and loose, remove it.* Observe her breathing. If your infant stops breathing, begin CPR. (See Breathing Emergency, page 53.)

12 If the object is not dislodged, give 2 breaths, 5 back blows, 5 chest thrusts, and then check for the object. Repeat this sequence until the object is dislodged or help arrives.

Caution:
• Do not try to dislodge and remove the object if you cannot see it.
• Never shake an infant to determine whether she is conscious.

Description: A life-threatening obstruction of the airway by an object, food, or croup.

What you need to know:	**When to get help:**
• If breathing has stopped, DO NOT begin emergency breathing until the airway is cleared.	• If someone is with you, call your local emergency number (911), while the other person follows the first-aid steps. • If you are alone, shout HELP! If you can do so quickly, call your local emergency number (911). Then follow the first-aid steps below. • Call your doctor for further instructions, even if you successfully dislodge the obstruction and your child seems fine.

Signs and symptoms:
• inability to breathe, cry, or make sounds
• high-pitched noises
• ineffective coughs
• bluish lips, nails, and skin

Treatment:
1 Stand behind your child and wrap your arms around his waist.

2 Make a fist with your hand. Grasp the fist with your other hand. Place the thumb-side of your fist in the middle of your child's abdomen, just above the navel and well below the tip of his breastbone.

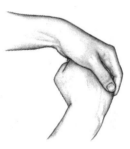

3 Keep your elbows out, and press your fist into your child's abdomen inward and upward with a series of 5 quick, distinct thrusts. Do not touch the breastbone or rib cage.

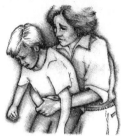

4 Continue these abdominal thrusts until the object is dislodged, help arrives, or your child loses consciousness. If your child loses consciousness, see the next section: Choking—For Unconscious Child Over 1 Year.

Caution:

• Do not interfere with your child if he can still cough, breathe, talk, or cry.

• Do not try to dislodge and remove the object if you cannot see it.

• Do not initiate first-aid steps until you are certain your child is actually choking. Encourage coughing to clear the airway. If your child can't cough, or if his cough is very weak, then follow the first-aid steps above.

Description: A life-threatening obstruction of the airway by an object, food, or croup.

What you need to know:	When to get help:
• If breathing has stopped, DO NOT begin emergency breathing until the airway is cleared.	• If someone is with you, call your local emergency number (911), while the other person follows the first-aid steps. • If you are alone, shout HELP! If you can do so quickly, call your local emergency number (911). Then follow the first-aid steps below. • Call your doctor for further instructions, even if you dislodge the obstruction and your child seems fine.

Signs and symptoms:
• inability to breathe, cry, or make sounds
• high-pitched noises
• ineffective coughs
• bluish lips, nails, and skin

Treatment:

1 Firmly supporting your child's head and neck, place her on her back onto a hard surface. Move your child as a unit, keeping her back in a straight line. Expose her chest.

2 Open your child's mouth with your thumb and index finger, placing your thumb over her tongue. *If the object is visible and loose, remove it with a hooked index finger.*

3 Look, listen, and feel for breathing. Lift your child's chin while tilting her head back to move her tongue away from her windpipe. Do not let her mouth close. Place your ear close to her mouth and watch for chest movement. For 5 seconds, look, listen, and feel for breathing.

4 If your child is not breathing, begin rescue breathing, as follows: Maintain her head position, close her nostrils by pinching them with your thumb and index finger, and cover her mouth tightly with your mouth. Give 2 slow, full breaths. Pause between the 2 breaths to take a deep breath.

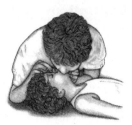

5 If you don't see her chest rise, reposition her head and give 2 more breaths.

6 If your child's chest still doesn't rise, begin abdominal thrusts, as follows: Kneel at her feet or astride her thighs. Place the heel of your hand in the middle of her abdomen just above her navel but well below the tip of her breastbone and rib cage. Place your other hand on top of the first hand.

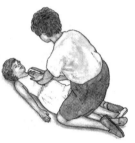

7 Press into your child's abdomen with a series of 5 quick, continuous upward thrusts.

8 Open your child's mouth with your thumb and index finger. *If the object is visible and loose, remove it with a hooked index finger.* Observe her breathing. If your child stops breathing, begin CPR:
—If your child is 1 to 8 years old, see Breathing Emergency—For Child Ages 1–8 Years, page 56.
—If your child is over 8 years old, see Breathing Emergency–For Child Over 8 Years, page 58.

9 If the object is not dislodged, give 2 breaths, 5 abdominal thrusts, and then check for the object. Repeat this sequence until the object is dislodged or help arrives.

Caution:
• Do not try to dislodge and remove the object if you cannot see it.

Description: A contagious infection of the nose and throat caused by many different viruses.

What you need to know:	**When to get help:**
• Colds are caused by viruses and do not require antibiotics. • Colds tend to be more contagious the day before symptoms appear and during the first 3–4 days.	• Call your doctor if: —Your child has difficulty breathing. —Your child has an earache or ear discharge. —Your child has a fever over 103°F. —Symptoms (especially fever) persist longer than 7 days.

Signs and symptoms:
• runny nose, congestion
• sore throat
• red, watery eyes
• cough
• fever
• decreased appetite

Treatment:
• Increase fluids; do not worry about solid food intake.
• Give acetaminophen or ibuprofen for fever.
• Use a nasal aspirator for congestion in infants.
• Use saline nose drops.
• Run a cool-air humidifier; keep it clean!

Caution:
• Avoid most over-the-counter cold medicines. Many have ingredients that may make your child jittery or prevent him from sleeping.

Related topics: Cough; Ear Infections; Laryngitis; Sinusitis

Description: Infection of the mouth (lips, corner of the mouth) caused by the herpes simplex virus.

What you need to know:	**When to get help:**
• Cold sores may spread throughout the mouth during *first* infection with this virus. • There is no specific treatment or prevention. • Cold sores may reappear with colds, fever, or stress. • Cold sores are not sexually transmitted. • They spread by close contact with someone who has the virus. • Sores may last 7–10 days. • They are a very common problem.	• Call your doctor if: —Your child refuses food and fluids for more than 24 hours. —Sores spread to the eyes. —Sores spread or worsen after one week. —Sores are accompanied by high fever over 103.5°F.

Signs and symptoms:
• burning, tingling before sores develop
• fever
• small blisters, ulcers

Treatment:
• Apply lip balm.
• Prevent picking.
• Use topical anesthetic (if recommended by your doctor).
• Give acetaminophen, ibuprofen.
• Increase liquids. (Your child may not want solid food.)
• Apply doctor-prescribed special solutions to sores.
• Avoid salty or acidic foods or hot liquids.

Related topics: Chicken Pox; Hand, Foot, and Mouth Disease

Description: Prolonged recurrent periods of intense crying with no apparent cause.

What you need to know:	**When to get help:**
• Colic frequently begins at about age 3 weeks and ends at about age 3 months. • The exact cause of colic is unknown. • The condition is rarely caused by sensitivity to milk (breast or formula).	• Call your doctor if: —You think your child has "colic," to eliminate more-serious causes. —Your soothing methods are ineffective.

Signs and symptoms:
• inconsolable crying spells (worse in the early evening)
• drawn up legs
• passing gas
• distended "stomach" (abdomen)

Treatment:
• Try various methods to calm your child:
  —rock her
  —carry her in a body carrier
  —supply a rhythmic motion or sound (music, vacuum cleaner)
  —rub her back
• Have someone watch the baby for an hour or two, and take a break if you are feeling stressed.
• If you are breastfeeding, try eliminating milk, caffeine, and potentially irritating foods from your diet. If these foods are the cause of your child's distress, symptoms should resolve in a few days.

Related topics: Constipation; "Stomach Pain" (Abdominal Pain)

Description: An injury to the brain caused by a fall or blow to the head.

What you need to know:	When to get help:
• Minor head injuries are inevitable in most children. • Scalp cuts or scrapes are common after head bumps.	• Call your doctor if: —You observe signs and symptoms indicating a significant injury (loss of consciousness, persistent vomiting, no improvement within a few hours, no memory of events preceding injury, blood coming from nose or ear). —Your child has a scalp cut that may need stitches. —Your child shows no improvement after a few hours of observation.

Signs and symptoms: (vary according to injury's severity and location)

Minor Head Injury
• dizziness
• nausea
• headache
• brief period of vomiting

Significant Head Injury
• persistent vomiting and/or headache
• confusion
• loss of consciousness
• no memory of events before accident
• bloody fluid from nose or ear
• convulsion

Treatment:
• Observe your child carefully; gradual improvement over 1–3 hours is the rule with minor injuries.
• Apply ice to scalp bleeding or swelling.
• If injury occurs in the evening, wake your child every 2 hours to be sure he can answer simple questions.

Description: Hard bowel movements.

What you need to know:	**When to get help:**
• One or more bowel movements a day is not a rule! Some children go every 2–3 days.	• Call your doctor if:
	—Constipation lasts for more than 1 week or recurs frequently despite home treatment.
• Constipation refers to the consistency of the stool, not the frequency.	—Blood is passed with stools.
• Brief periods of constipation are not uncommon in children.	—Your child shows signs of withholding stools.
• Observe for signs of resisting bowel movements (stool withholding).	—A potty-trained child begins soiling (leaking) stool in his underwear.

Signs and symptoms:
• dry, hard, and, often, less-frequent stools
• discomfort passing stools
• infrequent, large stools

Treatment:
• Have your child eat solid, high-fiber foods (whole-grain cereals, prunes, peas, bran).
• Do not give your child laxatives, suppositories, or enemas unless instructed by your doctor.

Related topics: "Stomach Pain" (Abdominal Pain)

Description: Sudden uncontrolled muscle movements or behavior changes caused by abnormal brain electrical activity.

What you need to know:

- Seizures themselves do not cause brain damage and are not life threatening unless prolonged (30–45 minutes).
- Most seizures in children over age 6 months and younger than 5 years result from fever and rarely last longer than 5–10 minutes.
- Protecting your child from injury during a seizure is essential.
- The term *epilepsy* refers to seizures without fever that recur over months or years.

When to get help:

- Call your doctor:
  —For any first seizure, with or without fever.
  —If your child experiences recurrent seizures, with or without fever.
- Call 911 if a seizure lasts longer than 5 minutes or breathing stops. (See Breathing Emergency, pages 53–59, depending on the child's age.)

Signs and symptoms:

- uncontrolled jerking, body movements
- rigid extremities
- pale, blue face and lips
- unresponsiveness
- rolled-back eyes
- drooling
- loss of bowel, bladder control

Treatment:

- Protect your child from injury.
- Call 911 if the seizure lasts longer than 5 minutes.
- Check the child's temperature after the seizure stops; if elevated, give acetaminophen or ibuprofen and call your doctor.

Related topics: Breath-Holding Spells; Encephalitis; Fever; Meningitis

Description: A symptom that occurs in response to an irritation in the air passages.

What you need to know:	**When to get help:**

• Cough is one of the body's defenses needed to clear the air passage of irritants; cough is good, not harmful!
 • In general, one does not want to suppress a cough.
 • Cough is a symptom, not a disease.
 • Some coughs indicate the source of the respiratory infection; most don't. For example, a barking cough usually originates from the larynx (voice box) and occurs with croup.
	• Call your doctor if:
	   —Your child is younger than 2–3 months of age.
	   —A fever of 103°F or higher is present.
	   —Your child has difficulty breathing.
	   —A cough persists longer than 10 days.
	 • Discuss with your doctor any questions you have regarding your child's need for cough medicines.

Treatment:
• Put a cool-air humidifier into your child's room.
• Increase liquids (to thin out mucus).
• Avoid cough medicines; they are generally not very helpful.
• If you use a cough medicine, do not use a medicine with multiple ingredients.
• Cough medicines with dextromethorphan (DM) may help if the cough is preventing your child from sleeping.

Related topics: Allergy; Asthma; Bronchitis; Cold; Croup; Whooping Cough (Pertussis)

Description: A condition resulting from increased "oil" production from sebaceous glands.

What you need to know:	**When to get help:**
• Cradle cap may spread to other areas of the body (face, creases of the neck, armpits, trunk, diaper area). • It is common in infants (younger than 3–4 months), and disappears at age 6 months to 1 year. • The rash causes no symptoms; it is not itchy.	• Call your doctor if: —Cradle cap does not improve in a week or two. —A rash develops in areas other than the scalp.

Signs and symptoms:
• oily, yellow scales
• scalp "dandruff"

Treatment:
• Shampoo your child's hair frequently with mild, baby shampoo or treatment recommended by your doctor.
• Use a soft brush or fine-toothed comb to remove scales.
• Use mineral oil or baby oil sparingly to loosen scales, and shampoo after use.

Related topics: Eczema; Ringworm

Description: Misalignment of the eyes caused by muscle imbalance.

What you need to know:
- Newborns and young infants can have periodic eye crossing.
- Some children appear to have crossed eyes because of certain facial structures (broad nasal bridge or folds of skin on either side of nose); this does not require specific treatment.

When to get help:
- Call your doctor if:
  —There is sudden onset of crossed eyes in your child after age 3 months.
  —Crossed eyes are present after age 4–6 months.

Signs and symptoms:
- eyes (one or both) turn in

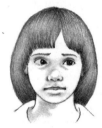

Treatment:
- If crossed eyes persist, your doctor will refer your child to an eye specialist.

Description: Inflammation and narrowing of area near the larynx (voice box) resulting in a barky cough.

What you need to know:	When to get help:
• Most croup is caused by viruses and requires no antibiotics. • Croup often begins suddenly at night and usually responds to home treatment.	• Call your doctor if: —The home remedies listed below do not produce a responce or if breathing difficulty worsens. —Your child has a temperature above 103°F. —Your child is unable to breathe comfortably and take liquids.

Signs and symptoms:
• barky, seal-like cough
• difficult, noisy breathing on inspiration (breathing in)
• fever
• hoarseness

Treatment:
• Run hot water in the bathroom shower to generate steam. Place your child in the steamed room for 15 minutes.
• If no improvement is seen after 15 minutes in the steam, take your child into the cool night air for 15 or 20 minutes.
• Give acetaminophen or ibuprofen for fever over 102°F.

Related topics: Allergy; Breathing Emergency; Cough; Diphtheria; Laryngitis

Description: Any break in the skin, such as abrasions (scrapes), lacerations, or punctures.

What you need to know:	When to get help:
• Most cuts can be handled at home. • Remain calm and your child is less likely to panic. • Evaluate wounds after bleeding stops and you've cleaned the area. • If the cut requires suturing, it should ideally be done within 8 hours, but can be done up to 18 hours; stitches reduce the size of the scar. • Antiseptics sting, and antibacterial ointment is generally unnecessary.	• Call your doctor if: —The wound is more than skin deep or longer than ½ to ¾ of an inch, or edges of cut separate. —Bleeding persists after 10–15 minutes of pressure. —Cut's edges are ragged or appear dirty. —Your child's tetanus immunization is incomplete. A booster is required if it has been 5 years since the previous inoculation. —Signs of infection (redness, swelling, fever) develop.

Treatment:

1 If the wound is bleeding, apply direct pressure with a clean cloth for 10 minutes.

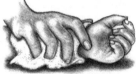

2 Wash the wound thoroughly. Use a turkey baster or syringe to flush out dirt.

3 If the bleeding is not profuse, apply ice in a plastic bag to minimize swelling. Otherwise, soak the wound in a tub.

4 Use a butterfly closure if it will approximate the wound edges. (See Bandages, page 24.)

5 Watch for signs of infection (redness, swelling, fever after 24 hours).

Related topics: "Blood Poisoning"

Description: An inherited disease that affects specific glands in many organs in the body.

What you need to know:	**When to get help:**
• Most problems in the lungs are due to blockage by excessively thick secretions. • Digestive problems are caused by a deficiency of digestive enzymes from the pancreas. • Both parents must be carriers of the gene for a child to get cystic fibrosis. • A gene abnormality recently has been detected. • Newer treatments have improved the outlook for children with cystic fibrosis. • Diagnosis of cystic fibrosis can be made with a sweat test (measures amount of salt on the skin).	• Call your doctor if the below signs and symptoms are present in your child. • If you have a family history of cystic fibrosis, discuss this with your doctor.

Signs and symptoms (depends on organ involved):
• poor growth rate
• chronic cough
• recurrent lung problems (pneumonia, wheezing)
• chronic diarrhea with foul-smelling, bulky stools

Treatment (depends on organ involved):
• Prescribed by your doctor after diagnosis is confirmed.
General Treatment
• Maintain good nutrition.
• Reduce lung infections and thin respiratory secretions.
• Replace pancreatic enzymes.

Related topics: Bronchitis; Diarrhea; Pneumonia

Description: The result of excessive loss of body fluids and salt.

What you need to know:	When to get help:
• Dehydration is commonly caused by diarrhea and vomiting. • Body fluids contain important salts and minerals that must be replaced when a child is dehydrated. • Clear liquids or various over-the-counter preparations (e.g., Pedialyte) replace lost fluids and salts; *they do not stop the vomiting or diarrhea.*	• Call your doctor if your child has vomiting or diarrhea and is unable to retain recommended liquids. • Call your child-care professional for feeding advice.

Signs and symptoms:
• listless (low energy level)
• dry mouth
• decreased tearing
• decreased urine output (fewer wet diapers)
• sunken eyes or soft spot
• wrinkled skin

Treatment:
• Follow feeding advice recommended by your health care professional. Call again if your child is not retaining fluids or if symptoms persist.

Related topics: Diabetes Mellitus; Diarrhea; Gastroenteritis; Heat Exhaustion; Heat Stroke; Vomiting

Description: A condition caused by lack of a hormone (insulin), resulting in the body's inability to process glucose (sugar) in the blood.

What you need to know:	When to get help:
• Insulin is produced in the pancreas, a gland located in the upper abdomen.	• Call your doctor if the below signs and symptoms are present in your child.
• Childhood diabetes (Type 1) is inherited; both parents must have the abnormal gene.	
• Type 2 diabetes occurs in adults and is not due to a total absence of insulin.	

Signs and symptoms:
• excessive and frequent urination
• excessive thirst/hunger
• weight loss
• fatigue

Severe Symptoms
• dehydration
• rapid breathing
• acetone odor to the breath

Treatment:
• Follow doctor-prescribed treatment regime—usually multiple insulin injections and special dietary instructions.

Related topics: Bedwetting; Dehydration

Description: A common irritation in the area covered by the diaper.

What you need to know:	**When to get help:**
• Most diaper rashes are not serious. It is a rare baby who does not get one at some time! • Diaper rashes are equally common in babies using cloth or disposable diapers. • Occasionally, the rash may be caused by a yeast infection (rash on thighs, abdomen) or bacteria (rash consists of small blisters or pustules).	• Call your doctor if: —Home treatment is unsuccessful after 4 days. —Blisters or pustules develop.

Signs and symptoms:
• redness, small red bumps, and small pimples

Treatment:
• Change diaper frequently.
• Wash area with mild soap; dry thoroughly.
• Apply zinc oxide or A & D ointment or other barrier creams.
• Expose diaper rash to air as much as possible.

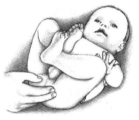

Description: Loose, often frequent bowel movements.

What you need to know:
- Common causes of diarrhea include gastroenteritis (see page 122) and drugs (especially antibiotics).
- If diarrhea is severe or prolonged, the body may lose important salts and water.
- Occasional loose bowel movements are common in children with upper respiratory infections (colds, sore throats, ear infections).
- Breast-fed babies normally have 5–10 loose bowel movements per day.

When to get help:
- Call your doctor if:
  —Your child has fever over 103°F, severe abdominal pain, or blood in the stool.
  —Diarrhea does not improve after 24 hours of home treatment.
  —Vomiting lasts more than 12 hours.
  —Your child has fever over 101°F for more than 48 hours.

Signs and symptoms:
- watery, green, or yellow stools
- abdominal cramping
- signs of dehydration (See Dehydration, page 96.)

Treatment:
- Continue your child's regular diet if your child has fewer than 5–6 loose bowel movements a day. The condition will resolve itself in a few days.
- Treat vomiting first, when it is present with diarrhea. Consult your doctor, or refer to Vomiting, page 208, for feeding instructions.
- Do not use over-the-counter diarrhea medicines, fruit juices, soda, or sports drinks (e.g. Gatorade).
- Give your child commercial electrolyte solutions (Pedialyte, Ricelyte) to replace lost salt and water. *These solutions do not stop diarrhea* and should not be used longer than 12–24 hours, unless instructed by your doctor.

Related topics: Cystic Fibrosis; Dehydration; Giardiasis; "Stomach Pain" (Abdominal Pain); Vomiting

Description: A bacterial infection that affects the respiratory system, nervous system, and heart.

What you need to know:	**When to get help:**
• Diphtheria is rare because of vaccination (DPT vaccine).	• Call your doctor if your child develops the below signs and symptoms, and your child is not immunized.
• The heart and muscle problems associated with diphtheria are caused by a toxin (poison) produced by the bacteria.	
• Your child should be immunized (at least three DPTs at ages 2 months, 4 months, and 6 months) and should have boosters at ages 15 months and 5 years.	
• Diphtheria is a serious, potentially fatal disease that requires hospitalization.	

Signs and symptoms:
• sore throat, gray plaque on throat and tonsils
• fever, headache, runny nose
• croupy cough
• heart failure, muscle paralysis

Treatment:
• There is no home treatment.

Related topics: Croup; Sore Throat (Pharyngitis, "Strep Throat"); Tonsillitis

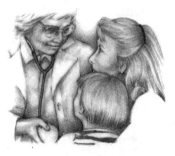

Description: The sensation that the body is unsteady or whirling around.

What you need to know:
- Dizziness results from a problem with the balancing mechanism located in the inner ear.
- Certain drugs, motion, or minor infection may cause dizziness.
- The most common cause of dizziness in children is the physical act of spinning around during play.

When to get help:
- Call your doctor if your child's dizziness:
  —Persists longer than 6–8 hours.
  —Recurs over hours or days.
  —Occurs after strenuous activity.

Signs and symptoms:
- loss of balance
- poor coordination
- lightheadedness
- nausea, vomiting occasionally

Treatment:
- Usually none is required.
- Have the child lie down or bend over for immediate relief.

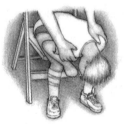

Related topics: Ear Infections; Fainting

Description: Suffocation by liquid, usually water, and possible hypothermia.

What you need to know:

• Give CPR if needed, even to a child who has been submerged for an extended period. Continue CPR until help arrives, or your child begins to breathe on her own.

If your child is under 1 year old, See Breathing Emergency for Infant under 1 Year, page 53.

If your child is 1 to 8 years old, See Breathing Emergency for Child Aged 1–8 Years, page 56.

If your child is over 8 years old, See Breathing Emergency for Child over 8 Years, page 58.

• With ice rescue, time is of the essence. Submersion in ice water can rapidly lead to hypothermia.

When to get help:

• Call your local emergency number (911) immediately, if possible.

• After an *ice rescue* call your local emergency number (911) if your child is unconscious, if she has been submerged for any period of time, if she is hypothermic (See Hypothermia, page 141), or if you have any concerns. Otherwise, call your doctor.

Treatment:

1 Have your child extend her arms flat on the ice and kick to keep afloat.

2 Kneel or lie down near the edge of the ice, brace yourself firmly, and reach for your child with your arm or an extended object, such as a stick, a rope, or clothing. If you must move onto the ice, lie flat and edge out slowly until the extended object is within the child's reach.

3 Have your child lie flat while you pull her to safety; don't let her get up and walk off the ice.

4 If you can't pull your child out with an extended object, and other people are available, form a human chain to pull her out. Have everyone slide out on the ice lying flat and spread-eagled, grasping the ankles of the person in front.

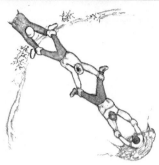

5 Observe your child's breathing, check the pulse, and give CPR if needed.

6 If your child vomits, turn her head to the side, and remove the vomitus from her mouth.

7 If your child is breathing, take her to a warm place, remove any wet clothing, wrap her in blankets, and call for professional help.

8 If your child is shivering uncontrollably, call your local emergency number (911) and treat her for possible hypothermia (See Hypothermia, page 141.)

Caution:
• Do not go out on the ice to rescue a child you can reach with your arm or an extended object.
• Do not let a drowning child grab you; she might pull you under.

Description: Suffocation by liquid, usually water.

What you need to know:	When to call for help:
• A child who is drowning often cannot call out for help. • Give CPR if needed, even to a child who has been submerged for an extended period. Continue CPR until help arrives or your child begins to breathe on his own. *If your child is under 1 year old,* See Breathing Emergency for Infant Under 1 Year, page 53. *If your child is 1 to 8 years old,* See Breathing Emergency for Child Aged 1–8 Years, page 56. *If your child is over 8 years old,* See Breathing Emergency for Child Over 8 Years, page 58.	• Call your local emergency number (911) immediately, if possible. • After a *water rescue* call your local emergency number (911) if your child is unconscious, if he has been submerged for any period of time, or if you have any concerns. Otherwise, call your doctor.

Treatment:

1 If your child is within reach, kneel or lie down near the edge of the water, brace yourself firmly, and reach for him with your arm or an extended object, such as a pole, oar, or towel.

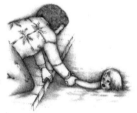

2 If your child is beyond reach, throw him a buoyant object, such as a board or life ring. If possible, throw an object with a line attached so you can pull him in; try to throw the object past him and then pull it within his reach. If the object has no line, tell your child to grab the object and kick to safety.

3 If your child is beyond reach, wade into the water if it is safe to do so, and extend an object to your child. Either pull your child to safety, or, if the object is buoyant, let go of it and tell your child to kick to safety. Be sure to keep the object between you and the child. Don't let him grab you.

4 If you must swim to your child, keep your eye on the spot where you last saw him, and bring an object for him to hold onto. Don't let him grab you.

5 If your child is not breathing, begin mouth-to-mouth resuscitation—while still in the water, if possible. Once on land, check the pulse and give CPR if needed. (See Breathing Emergency.)

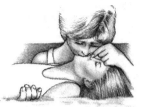

6 If your child vomits, turn his head to the side, and remove the vomitus from his mouth.

7 If your child is breathing, remove any wet clothing, wrap him in blankets, and call for professional help.

Caution:
• Do not enter the water to rescue a child who can be reached with your arm, a boat, an extended object, or a throwable object.
• Do not let a drowning child grab you. He might pull you under.

Description: Discharge from the ear canal resulting from infection or injury.

What you need to know:	When to get help:
• Never put anything "smaller than your elbow" into the ear. • Never try to remove a foreign object from the ear. • Blood flow from the ear may occur after a significant head injury. • Pus coming from the ear generally indicates an infection in the ear canal or a perforation of the ear drum from infection in the middle ear.	• Call your doctor if any discharge from the ear is noted.

Signs and symptoms:
• clear, yellow, or bloody discharge

Treatment:
• Treatment depends on the cause.

Description: Infected fluid in the middle ear (space behind the ear drum) caused by bacteria or viruses.

What to you need to know:	**When to get help:**

What to you need to know:
• Most ear infections (80–85 percent) resolve without treatment, but this cannot be predicted in the individual child. Therefore, all children should be treated.
• Ear infections are very common—two-thirds of all children will have at least one infection by age 2.
• Certain groups of children are more prone to develop ear infection (allergic children, children under age 1 in day care, certain ethnic groups—e.g., Native American).
• Initial treatment is usually with an antibiotic, and a follow-up is important to ensure that the fluid has cleared from the middle ear space.
• Persistence of fluid for long periods after treatment of the acute infection may result in hearing loss.

When to get help:
• Call your doctor if the below signs and symptoms are present, even if pain relief measures are effective. Resolution of pain does not mean the infection is resolved. An evaluation by your doctor is required.

Signs and symptoms:
• pain
• fever
• pulling ears
• waking from naps or night sleep
• ear discharge
• loss of balance
• cold symptoms (often precede an ear infection)

Treatment:
• Give acetaminophen or ibuprofen for pain.
• Administer ear drops (for pain) if prescribed by your doctor.
• Place your infant or child in an upright position to help relieve discomfort.

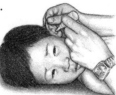

Related topics: Cold; Dizziness; Swimmer's Ear

Description: A chronic skin condition characterized by dry skin, itching, and a red, sometimes scaly, rash.

What you need to know:	When to get help:
• Scratching makes the rash worse; eczema is known as "the itch that rashes." • Some, but not all, children with eczema have other allergic disorders (asthma, hay fever). • Food elimination diets are rarely helpful. • Proper treatment of dry skin is the mainstay of treatment.	• Call your doctor if the rash is oozing (may be sign of infection) or not responding to home treatment.

Signs and symptoms:
• dry skin
• itchy, red rash on elbows, knees, and face of infants and in other areas in older children
• oozing sores, especially after scratching
• scaliness

Treatment:
• Use lubricating ointments for dry skin.
• Use Dove, Tone, or special cleansing agents recommended by your doctor.
• Pat dry after bathing; apply ointments while skin is still damp.
• Apply hydrocortisone cream or ointment if recommended by your doctor.
• Cut fingernails to reduce irritation from scratching.

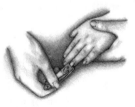

Related topics: Allergy; Asthma; Cradle Cap (Seborrhea)

Description: Severely reduced blood pressure (shock), unconsciousness, or burns resulting from contact with an electrical current.

What you need to know:	When to get help:
• An electrical shock may be brief and harmless, or it may be life threatening.	• Call your local emergency number (911) if your child is unconscious or has difficulty breathing. • Call your doctor if your child has electrical burns, which are often more severe than they seem.

Treatment:

• Unplug the cord or remove the fuse from the fuse box to turn off the electric current.

• If the current cannot be turned off, use a nonconducting object, such as a broom, chair, rug, or rubber doormat to push your child away from the source of the current. Do not use a wet or metal object. If possible, stand on something dry and nonconducting, such as a mat or folded newspapers.

• If your child has an electrical burn, remove any clothing that comes off easily and rinse the burned area in cool running water until the pain subsides. Use wet cloths to cover burned areas that cannot be immersed, such as the face. Pat dry.

• If the burn is still painful, cover the burned area with a clean, dry, nonfluffy dressing. If the burn is on your child's hand or foot, keep her fingers or toes apart by placing cloth or gauze between them; then loosely wrap the hand or foot in a clean dressing.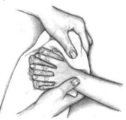

Caution:

• Do not touch your child with your bare hands while she is still in contact with the source of electricity.

• If burns are present, do not remove dead skin or break blisters.

• Do not apply ice, butter, ointments, medications, fluffy cotton dressings, or adhesive bandages to a burn.

Description: Inflammation of the brain tissue, usually secondary to an infection.

What you need to know:	**When to get help:**

• Encephalitis has many causes—the most common of which are different types of viruses.
• Other causes of encephalitis include insect-transmitted illnesses (e.g., Lyme disease).
	• Call your doctor if:
	   —The signs and symptoms below persist for any length of time.
	   —Hospitalization is required.

Signs and symptoms:
- headache
- fever
- vomiting
- stiff neck
- confusion
- lethargy
- convulsion

Treatment:
- There is no home treatment.

Related topics: Headaches; Meningitis; Vomiting

Description: A serious bacterial infection causing inflammation and blockage of the trachea (windpipe).

What you need to know:	When to get help:
• This infection has practically disappeared since the use of the Hib vaccine *(Hemophilus Influenza)*.	• Call your doctor if: —Your child has difficulty breathing and is drooling. —The usual home remedies (steam, increased humidity) do not produce a responce, and your child appears to have croup.

Signs and symptoms:
• fever
• sore throat
• difficulty swallowing
• harsh, noisy breathing
• drooling
• difficulty lying down
• child sits upright and leans forward

Treatment:
• Take your child into a room with a vaporizer or into a steam-filled bathroom.

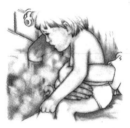

Related topics: Croup; Sore Throat (Pharyngitis, "Strep Throat")

Description: A blow or scratch to the eye.

What you need to know:	**When to get help:**
• You must be careful not to apply pressure to the cornea (the outer covering of the eyeball).	• Take your child to an emergency facility for a definitive diagnosis and medication, if needed, if your child's cornea is scratched.

Signs and symptoms:
• constant blinking of the eyes
• light sensitivity
• pain

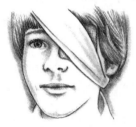

Treatment:
• Cover the affected eye with a clean dressing for 24–48 hours.
• Apply antibiotic drops if perscribed by your doctor.
• Have your doctor recheck the eye in 24 hours.

Caution:
• Do not let your child touch his eye.

Related topics: Bruise; Cuts, Wounds, Scrapes

Description: Burning of the eye with acid or alkali chemicals (battery acid, detergent, cleanser, etc.).

What you need to know:	When to get help:
• Prompt flushing of the eye is important.	• Take your child to an emergency facility if any chemicals get in your child's eye.

Treatment:

1 Turn your child's head so the injured eye is down and to the side. Holding the eyelid open, use a cup or a shower-head to pour water in the eye for 15 minutes (or use sterile eyewash).

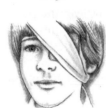

2 Cover the injured eye with a clean dressing, and don't let your child rub the injured eye.

Related topics: Bruise; Cuts, Wounds, Scrapes

Description: A cut of the eyelid or eyeball.

What you need to know:	**When to get help:**
• If a cut is large or turns black and blue, a tear duct or nerve may be injured, which requires professional treatment.	• Take your child to an emergency facility if the cut is large or turns black and blue.

Treatment:

1 If the cut is bleeding, apply direct pressure with a clean, dry cloth until the bleeding subsides.

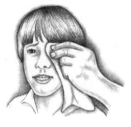

2 Clean the cut with water, cover with a clean dressing, and place a cold compress on the dressing to reduce pain and swelling.

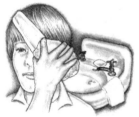

Related topics: Bruise; Cuts, Wounds, Scrapes

Description: Foreign objects (dust, dirt, gravel) in the eye; objects embedded in the eye.

What you need to know:	When to get help:
• Do not try to remove a foreign object that seems to be embedded in the eye. • Do not use sharp objects, such as tweezers, to remove the object.	• Take your child to an emergency facility if you cannot remove the foreign object (dirt, sand, and so on).

Treatment:

1 Grasp the top eyelid and pull it out and down over the eye. The object may wash out with tears.

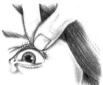

2 Gently depress the lower eyelid and look for the object. If you see the object, carefully lift it off with a clean cloth, or, if your child is cooperative, a cotton swab.

3 Have your child blink, which may force the object out.

4 If your child is cooperative, grasp his top eyelid and turn it back over a cotton swab. Have your child look down. Remove the object with a clean cloth or by flushing the eye with water or sterile eyewash.

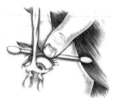

5 If the object cannot be removed, cover the eye with a clean dressing and call your doctor or take your child to an emergency facility.

Related topics: Bruise; Cuts, Wounds, Scrapes

Description: An abrupt, usually brief, loss of consciousness.

What you need to know:	When to get help:
• Fainting is caused by a temporary inadequate supply of oxygen to the brain. • Stress, fear, or pain may precipitate an event. • Spells usually last less than a minute.	• Call your local emergency number (911) if your child does not regain consciousness after 2 minutes, or if she begins jerking while unconscious (convulsion).

Signs and symptoms:
• light-headedness
• paleness
• dizziness
• sweating

Treatment:
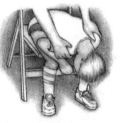
• If your child becomes light-headed, place her head between her knees.
• Loosen your child's clothing and make sure she has sufficient air.
• If your child loses consciousness, place her on her back and elevate her feet 8–12 inches. Do not place a pillow under your child's head.
• Turn your child's head to the side to prevent her from choking if she vomits.
• Wait 5–10 minutes after your child regains consciousness before allowing her to stand or walk. If she fell, check for any injuries. If you suspect significant injuries, especially to the head, call your doctor immediately.

Caution:
• Do not splash water on your child's face, shake her, or use smelling salts.

Related topics: Hyperventilation

Description: An oral temperature over 99.5°F or a rectal temperature above 100.4°F.

What you need to know:
- The main reason to treat fever is to make your child more comfortable. Children are rarely uncomfortable with a temperature below 102°F.
- Fever is not an illness; it is one of the body's means of fighting infection.
- Normal body temperature ranges from 97–100.4°F and varies depending on time of day (highest in late afternoon or early evening).
- If you think your child has a fever, take his temperature. Simply feeling your child's skin is inaccurate.
- Fevers do not cause brain damage.
- Convulsions (febrile seizures) occasionally occur and are rarely serious; however, this should warrant a call to your doctor.

When to get help:
- Call your doctor if:
  —Fever develops in a child under age 3 months.
  —Your child has fever over 104°F.
  —You are concerned about associated symptoms (earache, cough, and so on).
  —A convulsion occurs.

Signs and symptoms:
- body warm to the touch (not always reliable)
- flushed face
- chills
- sweating
- lack of energy

Treatment:
- Do not bundle a feverish child; dress him in cool clothing.
- Give acetaminophen or ibuprofen. (See dosage chart, pages 19–21.)
- Provide lukewarm-water sponge baths in a tub or basin if fever is over 104°F one hour after giving fever medicines.

Description: An infection caused by a virus, resulting in a characteristic rash.

What you need to know:	When to get help:
• Fifth disease is caused by Human Parvovirus B19 Virus (HPBV19).	• Call your doctor if you have questions about the contagiousness of this illness or for a specific diagnosis of the rash.
• This illness is most common in children ages 5–15 years.	
• A child is contagious before the rash develops, but not after.	
• The rash may come and go for weeks in some children, especially with sun exposure.	
• Fifth disease may cause severe anemia in children who have some underlying blood or immune diseases.	
• Children can go to school with the rash.	

Signs and symptoms:
• low-grade fever, malaise
• rash on cheeks (slapped-cheek appearance)
• lacy rash on extremities

Treatment:
• Treat fever with acetaminophen or ibuprofen. (See dosage charts, pages 19–21.)

Description: An injury to a fingertip causing intense pain, swelling, and black-and-blue fingernail.

What you need to know:	**When to get help:**
• Most fingertip tinjuries can be treated at home. • When a fingertip is injured, the nail may turn black and blue in several hours. Intense pain comes from accumulated blood trapped between nail and bone. Releasing the blood reduces the pain.	• Call your doctor if: —Bone deformity suggests fracture or dislocation. —Inability to straighten the finger suggests damage to tendon. —Treatment outlined below is impossible (child is uncooperative.) —Pain persists for hours after blood evacuation.

Treatment:

1 Apply ice or cold water as soon as possible to reduce swelling.

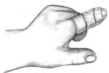

2 Heat a paperclip with a match. Hold the finger firmly in place and press down with the heated paperclip, as shown.

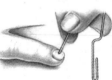

3 When nail is punctured, use gauze or cloth to absob the blood. Pain should be relieved within 20–30 minutes.

4 Cover the nail with gauze bandage, allowing the blood to continue to drain. Keep the nail covered for a few days.

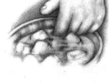

Related topics: Bruise; Cuts, Wounds, Scrapes

Description: Freezing of skin tissue and fluid as a result of exposure to extreme cold.

What you need to know:	When to get help:
• Frostbite most frequently affects exposed areas, such as the fingers, toes, ears, nose, and cheeks.	• Take your child to an emergency facility if you think that cold exposure was prolonged.

Signs and symptoms:
- numbness
- pain and burning
- hard skin
- yellowish-white or bluish-white skin
- blisters

Treatment:

1 Take your child indoors as soon as possible, remove wet clothing from the affected area, and remove any rings from frostbitten hands.

2 Immerse affected areas in warm (not hot) water—or apply warm cloths to affected ears, nose, or cheeks—for 20–30 minutes. Add water as needed to maintain water temperature. Your child probably will complain of intense pain as thawing progresses. After thawing, pat affected parts dry.

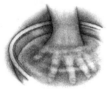

   —If feeling and color return, no further treatment is needed.
   —If feeling and color do not return, call your doctor and continue with Steps 3 through 5.

3 Wrap affected hands or feet loosely in a clean dressing. Keep fingers or toes apart by placing cloth or gauze between them before wrapping hands or feet. Be careful not to break blisters by rubbing.

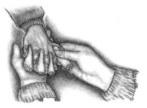

4 Elevate affected hands or feet. Have your child try to move the affected parts to increase circulation. Do not let her walk if her feet are affected.

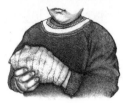

5 If the frostbite is extensive, give your child warm liquids to replace lost fluids.

Caution:
• Do not treat affected parts with hot water or a dry heat source, such as a hair dryer or space heater.
• Do not rub or massage affected parts or break blisters.
• Do not thaw affected parts if you are outdoors and refreezing could occur.

Related topics: Hypothermia

Description: Inflammation/infection of the digestive tract (stomach and intestines) most often caused by a virus, resulting in diarrhea with or without vomiting.

What you need to know:
• Rotovirus infection is the most common cause of gastroenteritis in young children.
• The symptoms last a few days to a few weeks.
• Careful attention to fluid intake and output is very important.
• Resuming a normal diet as soon as possible is essential.

When to get help:
• Call your doctor if:
—Blood is present in the vomitus or stool.
—Vomiting persists more than 12 hours.
—Abdominal pain is severe and persistent.
—Fever is greater than 104°.
—Your child shows signs of dehydration (see page 96).

Signs and symptoms:
• nausea/vomitting
• diarrhea
• abdominal cramps
• fever

Treatment:
• For vomiting, see page 208.
• For diarrhea, see page 99.
• If your child has fewer than 5 or 6 stools per day, continue his regular diet.
• Call your doctor for instructions about reintroducing solid foods if your child has been on Pedialyte (a commercial sugar and electrolyte solution used to replace lost salt and water) for more than 12 hours.

Related topics: Dehydration; Diarhhea; Fever; Vomiting

Description: A benign condition of the tongue characterized by painless white patches with red borders.

What you need to know:	**When to get help:**
• Geographic tongue is harmless, requires no treatment, and resolves in time. • There is a loss of papillae (taste buds) in the affected areas.	• Call your doctor if you have questions about the diagnosis.

Signs and symptoms:
• smooth patches of different colors, sizes, and shapes on the tongue

Treatment:
• None.

Description: A contagious viral disease characterized by mild constitutional symptoms and a red rash.

What you need to know:	When to get help:
• Infection with rubella early in pregnancy may result in abortion, stillbirth, or infants with congenital (birth) defects. • A vaccine (part of MMR—measles, mumps, rubella) is available for children at age 15 months. • A second vaccine is given at 5 years or 12 years of age. • Rubella is a mild infection, but is difficult to differentiate from many other common viruses.	• Call your doctor if your child is not immunized and you suspect rubella.

Signs and symptoms:
• low-grade fever (under 101°F)
• runny nose, followed by rash in 1–3 days
• swelling of glands behind ears and back of neck
• fine, red rash starting on face and spreading to trunk and extremities

Treatment:
• Give acetaminophen or ibuprofen for discomfort or temperature over 102°F. (See dosage charts, pages 19–21.)

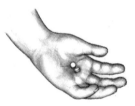

Description: An infection of the small intestine caused by a parasite.

What you need to know:	When to get help:
• The disease may be spread from other children or from contaminated food or water. • Symptoms are generally mild, but if untreated, may cause prolonged diarrhea and weight loss.	• Call your doctor if diarrhea does not resolve in a week or is unresponsive to the usual home remedies.

Signs and symptoms:
• nausea
• abdominal pain
• bloating (increased gas)
• diarrhea, foul-smelling stools
• weight loss

Treatment:
• Administer prescribed treatment once diagnosed.

Related topics: Diarrhea; "Stomach Pain" (Abdominal Pain)

Description: An enlarged thyroid gland.

What you need to know:	When to get help:
• Symptoms may be related to an overactive or underactive thyroid gland. • Tests are required to determine the cause of the goiter.	• Call your doctor if you notice swelling in the center of the neck.

Signs and symptoms:
• swelling in the center of the neck around the "Adam's apple"

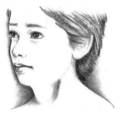

Treatment:
• Depends on the specific diagnosis.

Description: A viral infection that causes lesions in the mouth and on the hands and/or feet.

What you need to know:	When to get help:
• A child with hand, foot, and mouth disease generally is not sick. • The disease lasts a few days and requires no treatment.	• Call your doctor if diagnosis is uncertain.

Signs and symptoms:
• blisters in mouth and on hands and feet
• low-grade fever

Treatment:
• Provide fever measures for discomfort or temperature over 102°F.
• Avoid spicy foods and citrus and carbonated beverages—they may irritate the blisters in the mouth and may be painful to eat or drink.
• Give your child cool liquids and Popsicles to soothe the irritation.

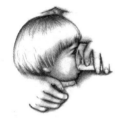

Related topics: Blister; Cold Sore (Fever Blister)

Description: Allergic disorder resulting in nose and eye inflammation.

What you need to know:	When to get help:
• Allergic inflammation of the nose may be caused by any allergenic substance (dust, animal dander, and so on). • Symptoms in fall or spring are often caused by grasses or pollens (especially ragweed in the fall).	• Call your doctor if the below signs and symptoms persist or recur at the same time each year.

Signs and symptoms:
• nose congestion, clear discharge
• sneezing
• red, itchy eyes with increased tearing

Treatment:
• Administer prescribed treatment, medicine, and recommended environmental control measures, such as reducing the child's exposure to dust and pollen (e.g., keeping the windows closed and using air conditioning during the summer, frequent vacuuming of child's carpet, and so on).

Related topics: Allergy; Asthma; Eczema

Description: Scalp infestation caused by small insects, resulting in irritation and itching.

What you need to know:
- Lice are spread by personal contact or by objects, such as combs or brushes.
- The incidence of this very common problem is increasing among school-aged children.
- Eggs (nits) appear as whitish flecks on the hair shaft and cannot easily be brushed away like dandruff.

When to get help:
- Call your doctor if:
  —You suspect lice but need confirmation.
  —Home treatment fails, or the problem recurs.

Signs and symptoms:
- scalp itching
- scalp inflammation, irritation secondary to scratching
- small, grayish-white eggs (nits) seen on hair shaft
- enlarged lymph glands in back of neck

Treatment:
- Use RID or NIX. (Directions for use are on the package.)
- Treat all household members; for pregnant women and infants under age 2 months, consult your doctor.

Description: Localized or generalized pain resulting from multiple causes.

What you need to know:	**When to get help:**
• Most children at some time complain of headaches, which are either insignificant or self-limited and respond to treatment with mild analgesics (pain relievers). • Some causes of headaches include stress, high blood pressure, migraine, head injury, and infection.	• Call your doctor if: —Your child's headaches are recurrent or unresponsive to home treatment. —The headaches occur when your child seems quite ill (high fever, vomiting, lethargy).

Signs and symptoms:
• may be described as a "dull ache," throbbing, constant, or intermittent pain
• may occur in one location or be generalized
• may manifest in infants by fussiness, irritability, or excessive crying

Treatment:
• Give acetaminophen or ibuprofen. (See dosage charts, pages 19–21.)
• Massage the child's head and/or neck.

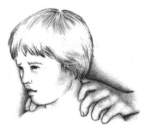

Related topics: Encephalitis; Meningitis; Sinusitis; Sore Throat (Pharyngitis, "Strep Throat")

Description: A condition that occurs when the body overheats due to excessive heat in the environment and/or overexertion.

What you need to know:	When to get help:
• Heat exhaustion is not a medical emergency, but does require prompt attention. • It can follow normal exertion in a hot environment or overexertion in moderate temperatures. • Heat exhaustion is different than heat stroke.	• Call your doctor if your child's temperature is above 101°F, or if signs or symptoms last longer than 1–2 hours or worsen. • Call your local emergency number (911) if your child's temperature is high— 102–106°F.

Signs and symptoms:
• fatigue
• nausea
• dizziness
• profuse sweating
• thirst
• normal or slightly elevated temperature

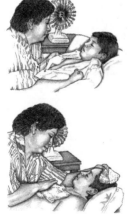

Treatment:
• Remove your child from sunlight and have him lie down in a cool place. Loosen his clothing.
• Unless your child is vomiting, have him sip water or juices every 10–15 minutes.
• Apply cool, wet cloths to your child's skin and fan him.

Related topics: Heat Stroke

Description: Rash caused by a blockage of the sweat glands, often on neck and upper chest, especially on newborns.

What you need to know:	When to get help:
• Heat rash is common and not serious.	• Call your doctor if: —Rash persists despite home treatment. —Other symptoms develop, which may mean the rash is caused by something other than heat.

Signs and symptoms:
• small, red bumps noted in the following areas: cheeks, neck, behind the ears, and diaper area
• occurs in warm weather if baby is overdressed; detergents and bleaches may aggravate the rash

Treatment:
• Do not overdress your child. Keep her skin cool and dry.
• Do not use oily skin products. (They may block pores.)
• Use baby powder in very small amounts. 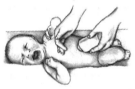 (Use carefully. Do not shake the container vigorously; baby should not inhale the powder.)

Description: A life-threatening condition due to a failure of the body's temperature-regulating ability, caused by extreme heat.

What you need to know:	**When to get help:**
• Heat stroke can be very serious. It can be fatal if not treated promptly.	• Call your local emergency number (911) if you suspect heat stroke, and immediately try to lower your child's body temperature.

Signs and symptoms:
• absence of sweating
• hot, flushed skin
• headache
• dizziness, confusion, loss of consciousness
• nausea/vomiting
• muscle cramps
• bounding, or weak and rapid pulse
• high temperature (102–106°F).

Treatment:
• Remove your child from direct sunlight and do one of the following cool-down procedures:

—Place your child in a tub of cool (not cold) water up to his navel, and rub a wet washcloth or towel over his body.

—Put your child in a cool shower or under a garden hose.

—Lay your child in a cool room in front of a fan or air conditioner, and wrap him in wet sheets or towels.

Continue cooling your child until his temperature drops to 102°F or lower.

• When your child's temperature has dropped to 102°F, pat him dry, lay him down, and cover him with a dry sheet. Fan him or put him in front of a fan or air conditioner. If his temperature begins to rise, repeat the cool-down procedure.

Caution:
• Do not give your child medications or stimulants such as caffeinated soft drinks.

Related topics: Fever; Heat Exhaustion

Description: Inflammation of the liver, most often caused by viruses.

What you need to know:	When to get help:
• There are various types of viral hepatitis, and they differ in their mode of transmission. • Hepatitis A (most common in children) is mild and often goes undetected because no jaundice is present. • Immunization against hepatitis B is recommended for infants. • Immunization against hepatitis A is available when indicated, but is not recommended routinely. • Hepatitis is most often spread by another person or acquired through blood transfusions. • Children who become jaundiced are contagious for 1 week after symptoms subside.	• Call your doctor if your child has been exposed to someone with hepatitis or to someone who has the below signs and symptoms.

Signs and symptoms:
• loss of appetite and malaise
• nausea, vomiting
• abdominal pain (upper abdomen)
• jaundice (green- and yellow-colored skin and white of the eyes; rarely occurs in children)
• dark urine

Treatment:
• Wash hands after changing your child's diaper and before preparing food to prevent the spread of hepatitis.
• Teach older children to wash their hands after bowel movements.

Related topics: Jaundice (in newborns); Anemia (in older children)

Description: A protrusion of tissue (usually intestine) through a weak spot in the abdomen.

What you need to know:	**When to get help:**
• Hernias of the umbilicus often resolve without treatment by age 4–5.	• Call your doctor if:
• Hernias in the groin or scrotum require surgical treatment.	—You observe a possible hernia in your child.
	—Your child has pain, and the hernia will not reduce with a gentle push.

Signs and symptoms:
• bulging groin, umbilicus (navel) that may persist or appear when the child cries or strains
• scrotum bulge in boys

Treatment:
Umbilical Hernia
• Observation.
Inguinal (groin) Hernia
• Surgery.

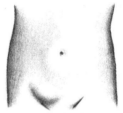

Related topics: Testicle, Torsion

Description: Infection caused by Type 1 or Type 2 herpes viruses.

What you need to know:	**When to get help:**
• Type 2 herpes is sexually transmitted. • Babies born to mothers with herpes can contract the disease during birth. If a pregnant woman has active lesions or a history of herpes, she should inform her doctor. • The first episode of Type 1 herpes spreads throughout the inside of the mouth. • After the first episode, the virus remains in the body in a latent (dormant) form, and certain triggers (e.g., stress, colds) reactivate the virus, resulting in "cold sores" around the lips.	• Call your doctor if: —Diagnosis is unclear. —Diagnosis is clear, and child refuses fluids longer than 12–18 hours.

Signs and symptoms:

Oral Herpes (Type 1)
• painful blisters (ulcers) on mouth
Genital Herpes (Type 2)
• blisters on genital area

Treatment:
• Offer clear liquids, milk shakes.
• Give acetaminophen or ibuprofen.
• Rinse mouth with a mixture prescribed by your physician.
• Treat genital herpes with a special prescription medicine.

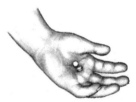

Related topics: Cold Sore (Fever Blister); Hand, Foot, and Mouth Disease

Description: A specific allergic reaction of the skin characterized by itchy "welts."

What you need to know:	When to get help:
• Hives can be caused by medications, minor infections, and certain foods (nuts, chocolate).	• Call your doctor if:
	—The itching makes your child uncomfortable.
• In most cases, the cause of hives cannot be identified.	—Your child has trouble breathing.
• Most cases of hives resolve in a few days.	
• Hives may result from an insect bite (e.g., bee sting).	

Signs and symptoms:
• raised, itchy welts (large blisters) of varying sizes that come and go

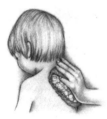

Treatment:
• Give oral antihistamines.
• Apply cool compresses (or give a cool bath).

Related topics: Allergy; Bites, Stings (Animal, Human, Snake)

Description: Developmental disorder that affects children's behavior and learning.

What you need to know:	When to get help:
• Hyperactivity may be the result of many underlying problems, not only ADHD. • If your child is hyperactive, a thorough evaluation conducted by your child's physician or other specialist is required. • ADHD is most often diagnosed when a child enters school and has difficulty learning.	• Call your doctor if your child has some of the below signs and symptoms.

Signs and symptoms:
• easily distracted
• difficulty concentrating
• impulsivity
• easily frustrated
• mood swings
• learning problems

Treatment:
• Schedule a thorough evaluation by a competent professional in this field to determine the cause of your child's hyperactivity.
• If ADHD is diagnosed and treatment is recommended, administer medication as prescribed by your physician.

Description: The sensation of "air hunger" causing over-breathing, usually a result of anxiety.

What you need to know:	When to get help:
• Anxiety is the usual underlying cause of hyperventilation. • Tingling, numbness, and muscle spasms are caused by blowing off too much carbon dioxide. • Hyperventilation occurs most often in older children and teenagers.	• Call your doctor if symptoms persist or occur frequently.

Signs and symptoms:
• rapid breathing, sensation of "air hunger"
• numbness, tingling in hands and feet
• muscle spasms
• fainting

Treatment:
• Reassure your child.
• Have your child breathe into a paper bag for 5 or 10 minutes.
• Schedule a complete evaluation to determine the underlying cause of anxiety.

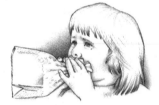

Related topics: Fainting

Description: A disorder in which the level of glucose (sugar) in the blood is low.

What you need to know:	**When to get help:**
• Hypoglycemia is a symptom, not a disease. • There are many possible causes of hypoglycemia; therefore, a complete medical evaluation is necessary.	• Call your doctor if: —You suspect hypoglycemia based on the above symptoms, especially if symptoms are recurrent. —Diagnosis has been confirmed by a blood test for glucose. *(This is the only definitive way to make the diagnosis.)*

Signs and symptoms:
- paleness
- headache
- drowsiness
- irritability
- sweating
- dizziness, fainting
- convulsions

Treatment
• After a medical evaluation has been completed, follow the treatment prescribed by your doctor.

Related topics: Headaches; Convulsion

Description: Severe heat loss leading to dangerously low core body temperatures.

What you need to know:	When to get help:
• Bodies lose heat much faster in cold water or through wet clothing than when dry.	• Call your local emergency number (911) if you observe the signs and symptoms listed below, if your child's temperature is less than 95°F, or if you think that cold exposure was prolonged.

Signs and symptoms:
- uncontrollable shivering
- weakness
- drowsiness
- confusion
- slowing of breathing
- shock

Treatment:
• Bring your child into a warm room (if in the woods, start a fire and create shelter from the wind), remove any wet clothing, and keep your child awake.
• Wrap your child in warm blankets or clothing and cover her head; then apply heat to her torso with hot-water bottles or heating pads, and/or warm her with body-to-body contact.
• If your child is conscious, give her warm liquids.

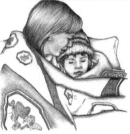

Related topics: Frostbite

Description: Bacterial infection of the skin.

What you need to know:	**When to get help:**
• Impetigo is a contagious condition caused by staph and strep bacteria. • Rarely, kidney problems (acute nephritis) may result if impetigo is caused by certain strains of strep.	• Talk to your doctor if you suspect your child has impetigo.

Signs and symptoms:
• yellowish (pus-filled) blisters
• weeping skin sores
• scabs, crusted lesions

Treatment:
• Give warm soaks to loosen and remove pus.
• If only a few sores are present, apply antibiotic ointment (Bactroban), as prescribed by your physician.
• If the condition is more extensive, administer oral antibiotic treatment for 10 days.

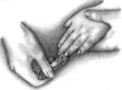

• Clip your child's nails to discourage scratching, as this spreads the disease.

Related topics: Blister

Description: A common viral infection of the respiratory tract that occurs during the winter months.

What you need to know:
- Influenza is very contagious, frequently occurs among many members of a community, and is spread by respiratory secretions.
- Many different strains of the influenza virus (Type A, Type B) can be predicted before the "flu season"; thus, a different vaccine is available each year.
- The disease lasts about a week.
- Antibiotics are not indicated for flu.

When to get help:
- Call your doctor if:
  —You observe no improvement after 5–6 days.
  —Your child develops breathing difficulty.

Signs and symptoms:
- fever, chills
- cough
- muscle aches
- headache
- poor appetite

Treatment:
- *DO NOT give your child aspirin.* (It may cause Reye's syndrome.)
- Give acetaminophen or ibuprofen. (See dosage charts, pages 19–21.)
- Increase fluids; get plenty of bed rest.
- Offer cough medicines at night, if recommended by your health care professional.

Related topics: Cough; Headaches; Pneumonia; Reye's Syndrome

Description: Redness, pain, and swelling caused by an incorrectly cut toenail that irritates nearby skin.

What you need to know:	**When to get help:**
• The large toenail is most often involved. • Ingrown toenails are usually caused by cutting toenails improperly at the edge or by wearing excessively tight shoes	• Call your doctor if: —Signs of infection (pus, red streaks) occur. —The condition fails to improve with home treatment.

Signs and symptoms:
• redness, pain, and swelling, usually on one side of the nail.

Treatment:
• Apply warm soaks.
• Gently lift the corner of the nail and wedge a small piece of cotton under it; repeat frequently until the nail grows enough to be trimmed.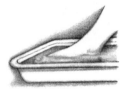
• Cut toenails straight across, leaving the ends of nails slightly longer; be sure that shoes fit properly.

Description: A sign, not a disease, caused by an increase in a substance (bilirubin) in the blood, resulting in a yellow-green tinge to the skin, mucus membranes, and whites of eyes.

What you need to know:	When to get help:
• Jaundice in newborns after 24 hours is very common, especially in breast-fed babies, and is rarely serious. Jaundice in newborns may last for a few weeks to a month. • Jaundice in older infants or children is always significant and requires a physician's evaluation.	• Call your doctor if jaundice in your newborn: —Increases after 5–7 days. —Develops after your newborn leaves the hospital. —Is accompanied by signs of illness (poor feeding, inactivity, low or elevated temperature).

Signs and symptoms:
• yellow-green discoloration of skin and whites of eyes

Treatment:
• Follow regimen as prescribed by your physician after a specific cause is determined.

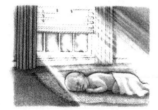

Related topics: Anemia; Hepatitis

Description: An inflammation of the vocal cords causing hoarseness.

What you need to know:	When to get help:
• Laryngitis is usually caused by a virus and is self-limited (no specific treatment). • It is often accompanied by cold symptoms.	• Call your doctor if: —Laryngitis is associated with high fever (over 103°F). —Breathing difficulty develops. —Hoarseness lasts longer than 1 week.

Signs and symptoms:
- hoarseness, loss of voice
- runny nose, cough
- possible fever

Treatment:
- Give acetaminophen or ibuprofen for fever over 102°F. (See dosage charts, pages 19–21.)
- Have your child rest his voice (if possible).
- Keep room humidified.

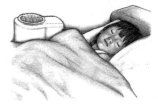

Related topics: Croup; Epiglottitis

Description: Pain in the lower leg that occurs at night.

What you need to know:	**When to get help:**
• Growing pains almost always occur at night and may awaken your child. • Pain generally occurs in the shin area. • The cause of leg pain is unknown, but probably is related to vigorous activity and has nothing to do with your child's growth.	• Call your doctor if: —Pain occurs when your child is awake. —Swelling occurs in your child's legs or joints.

Signs and symptoms:
• muscle aches, usually in both lower legs

Treatment:
• Apply heat; massage.
• Give acetaminophen or ibuprofen.
(See dosage charts, pages 19–21.)

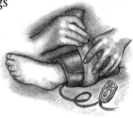

Description: Cancer of the white blood cells.

What you need to know:	When to get help:
• Leukemia, although uncommon, is one of the most common childhood cancers.	• Call your doctor if you suspect your child may have leukemia because of the below signs and symptoms.
• Approximately 80 percent of children with the most common type of leukemia (lymphocytic) can be cured.	
• The prognosis continues to improve for patients with leukemia with the development of new drugs and new drug-combination therapies.	

Signs and symptoms:
• paleness (secondary to anemia)
• fever
• swollen lymph nodes
• joint or bone pain
• spontaneous bruising or bleeding
• enlarged spleen and liver

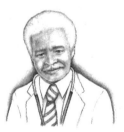

Treatment:
• Managed by a cancer specialist.

Related topics: Anemia; Swollen Lymph Glands

Description: Bacterial infection transmitted by deer ticks.

What you need to know:
- It is called *Lyme disease* because the first cases were diagnosed in Lyme, Conn.
- The disease is caused by the deer tick, which is much smaller than the common wood tick.
- The tick must remain on the skin at least 48 hours before it can cause the disease.
- The long-term complications (joint, nervous system, heart) can be prevented with early detection and treatment.
- Lyme disease occurs most often in the summer and fall, and is most common in the Midwest and Northeast.

When to get help:
- Call your doctor if:
  —You notice the lesion described below.
  —You suspect your child has symptoms of Lyme disease.

Signs and symptoms:
- circular, expanding rash that clears in center (Erythema Migrans)
- "flu-like" symptoms (fever, fatigue, headache, muscle aches)

Treatment:
- Take preventative measures:
  —Have your child wear a hat, a long-sleeved shirt, and long pants tucked into boots if hiking in the woods.
  —Dress your child in light-colored clothing to detect ticks easier.
  —Inspect for ticks carefully (especially behind the ears and at the hairline).
  —Do not use products containing DEET on infants.
- Remove a tick by grasping with tweezers close to the skin, or with a finger protected by tissue, and gently pulling straight out; try to avoid crushing the tick. Crushing would cause more material to be injected into the skin. Store the tick in a glass container in case your doctor needs to see it.
- Treat signs and symptoms of Lyme disease early with antibiotics to cure the disease and prevent complications.

Related topics: Arthritis

Description: A highly contagious viral infection characterized by fever, respiratory symptoms, red eyes, and a characteristic rash.

What you need to know:	**When to get help:**

• Measles is preventable with immunizations (MMR) given at ages 15 months and at 5 years or 12 years.
• Immunization is essential because complications from the disease can be serious or fatal.
	• Call your doctor if:
	  —Your child is unimmunized and you suspect measles.
	  —An unimmunized infant (less than age 15 months) is exposed to measles.

Signs and symptoms:
• fever
• hacking cough
• red eyes
• white spots inside of cheeks (Koplik spots)
• rash (appearing 3–5 days after "cold" symptoms, starting on the face/neck, and spreading to the rest of the body)

Treatment:
• Prevent measles by immunization.
• There is no specific treatment for a measles infection.

Description: Inflammation of the membranes surrounding the brain and spinal cord (meninges) caused by various infectious organisms (bacteria, viruses).

What you need to know:	When to get help:
• Meningitis is a serious disease and requires early detection and treatment to prevent complications. • Some forms are highly contagious.	• Call your doctor if you suspect your child has meningitis based on the below signs and symptoms.

Signs and symptoms:
• fever (often high, 104°F)
• headache
• vomiting
• lethargy
• stiff neck

Treatment:
• Hospitalization and antibiotic treatment are required for bacterial meningitis.

Related topics: Encephalitis; Headaches; Vomiting

Description: Irregular menstrual periods and/or flow in the early years of menstruation.

What you need to know:	**When to get help:**
• Menstruation generally begins in girls between ages 8–9 and 17 years (average age 12). • It may take months or years for regular periods to occur because of hormone imbalance.	• Call the doctor if your daughter's periods: —Begin before age 8–9 or have not occurred by age 16. —Are extremely heavy or painful. —Stop for longer than 4 months.

Signs and symptoms:
- abdominal cramps
- backache
- headache
- irregular periods
- light or heavy flow

Treatment:

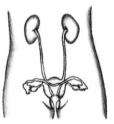

- Discuss menstruation with your daughter to remove any misconceptions.
- Provide books on menstruation for your daughter to read.
- Give ibuprofen for severe cramps.

Description: Round pigmented (brown, black) growths on the skin.

What you need to know:	When to get help:
• Almost everyone has a few moles that appear in childhood or adolescence. • Most moles are benign. • If a mole, with or without hair, is present at birth, consult your physician.	• Call your doctor if the mole increases rapidly, bleeds frequently, or changes color or shape. • Discuss with your doctor moles that are present at birth.

Signs and symptoms:
• small brown, black, or flesh-colored spots or lumps that occasionally are hairy or wart-like
• some moles have a halo (clear area) surrounding them

Treatment:
• Treatment is usually not required.
• Have moles surgically removed, under special circumstances, per your physician's recommendation.

Related topics: Birthmarks

Description: Skin infection characterized by raised, smooth, waxy nodules with an indented center.

What you need to know:	**When to get help:**
• The disease is spread by contact with an infected person. • Most cases will resolve without specific treatment.	• Call your doctor if you suspect molluscum contagiosum in your child.

Signs and symptoms:
• one or many round, raised, waxy pimples with an indented center (resembling miniature volcanoes)

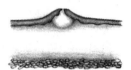

Treatment:
• There are various treatments available (freezing, destroying each lesion with a special tool, special cream) as recommended by your doctor.
• Limit contact between infected child and family members to prevent spread of infection.
• Keep the infected child's clothing, towels, and bedding separate until laundering, which kills the virus.

Description: A viral infection usually characterized by fever, sore throat, and enlarged lymph nodes.

What you need to know:	When to get help:
• Children under age 5 rarely have the typical symptoms of mononucleosis and the usual office tests are rarely positive; thus, the disease is infrequently diagnosed. • Some children under age 5 have had mononucleosis, but with few or no symptoms. • There is no specific treatment. • The virus of infectious mononucleosis is transmitted from mouth secretions ("kissing disease"). • Infectious mononucleosis can be diagnosed with special blood tests.	• Call your doctor if your child has been diagnosed with infectious mononucleosis and develops drooling or breathing difficulty.

Signs and symptoms:

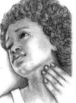

- fever
- sore throat
- malaise
- swollen lymph glands

Treatment:
- Administer acetaminophen or ibuprofen for fever. (See dosage charts, pages 19–21.)
- Offer throat lozenges for sore throat.
- Limit your child's activity if recommended by your doctor.
- Restrict your child's participation in contact sports to reduce the chance of possible spleen injury, if recommended by your doctor.

Related topics: Headaches; Sore Throat (Pharyngitis, "Strep Throat"); Tonsillitis

Description: A disorder caused by repetitive movement (car, swing) characterized by nausea and/or vomiting.

What you need to know:	When to get help:
• Some children are more predisposed than others to motion sickness; it is not the child's fault.	• Call your doctor if: —Your child has a history of motion sickness and may require treatment. —Persistent vomiting develops.

Signs and symptoms:
- nausea
- vomiting
- pallor
- cold sweating

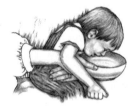

Treatment:

• Position your child where there is the least motion (car—front seat; airplane—over wing; boat—rear seat).

• Have your child look forward in transit, not to the side.

• Have your child avoid reading while in transit.

• Administer a special medicine, which is given 1 hour before a trip, as prescribed by your doctor.

Description: Injury to the teeth, lips, or tongue.

What you need to know:	When to get help:
• Prompt treatment is important. • Cuts of the lip and tongue may, or may not, need sutures.	• Call your doctor if your child has lip or tongue lacerations (cuts). • Call your local emergency number (911) or take your child to an emergency facility if bleeding cannot be controlled. • Call your dentist immediately if *permanent* teeth are loosened or cracked; *primary* teeth are less important, since they will fall out anyway.

Signs and symptoms:
• bleeding
• swelling
• loose, chipped, or dislodged tooth
• cut

Treatment:
• Place broken or dislodged permanent teeth in milk, and call your dentist immediately.
• Apply immediate pressure (with a clean cloth) for 5–10 minutes until bleeding stops.
• Have your child sit upright to minimize swelling and bleeding.

Description: Contagious viral disease characterized by swelling of the salivary glands (most often the parotid).

What you need to know:	**When to get help:**
• Mumps is uncommon today because of immunization (MMR) given at age 15 months and at 5 years or 12 years. • When swelling of the parotid glands occurs in an immunized child, it is usually due to another virus, or some other cause. • Children under 1 year are generally immune to mumps.	• Call your doctor if: 　—You need to diagnose the cause of swelling noted in front of the ear. 　—Your child has mumps and develops a severe headache and/or vomiting.

Signs and symptoms:
• swelling in front of the ears, on one or both sides
• low-grade fever
• malaise

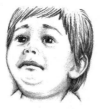

Treatment:
• Provide fever and pain treatment—acetaminophen, ibuprofen.
• Avoid acidic substances (e.g., orange juice).

Description: An inflammation of the kidney resulting from multiple causes.

What you need to know:	**When to get help:**
• There are many causes of nephritis. Laboratory tests are required to make a specific diagnosis. • A form of nephritis in children occurs in 2–4 weeks following a strep infection of the throat.	• Call your doctor if the below signs and symptoms are present in your child, especially if you notice color changes in the urine.

Signs and symptoms:
• headache
• poor appetite
• puffy eyes (especially on awakening)
• red or cola-colored urine

Treatment:
• Follow your doctor's recommendations.

Related topics: Headaches; Impetigo; Sore Throat (Pharyngitis, "Strep Throat")

Description: "Scary" dreams that occur most often in the early-morning hours.

What you need to know:	When to get help:
• Children vividly describe dreams, which are often remembered the following day, and may resist going back to sleep. • Nightmares may occur with increasing frequency during times of stress or with fever. • Nightmares are different than night terrors, which occur earlier in the sleep cycle (midnight), are not recalled the following day, and are associated with sleepwalking.	• Call your doctor if nightmares increase in frequency, are associated with stressful situations, or you think your child may be having night terrors.

Signs and symptoms:
• sudden waking
• fearfulness

Treatment:
• Reassure your child constantly.
• Discuss nightmares with your child.
• Seek professional counseling if required.

Description: Injury to the nose causing bleeding.

What you need to know:	When to get help:
• Dry air, vigorous blowing, nosepicking, and injuries to the nose cause most nosebleeds.	• Call your doctor if bleeding persists after 15–20 minutes of treatment, if nosebleeds recur, or if blood persistently drains down your child's throat.

Signs and symptoms:
• blood coming from nose
• blood in throat or vomit (bleeding from nose drains into throat)

Treatment:

1 Calm and reassure your child. Bleeding will be less severe if she relaxes.

2 Have your child lean forward. Pinch her nose shut for at least 10 minutes to allow a blood clot to form. Do not let your child sniff or blow her nose for several hours. If the bleeding persists or recurs, repeat the pinching.

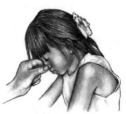

3 After the bleeding stops, gently apply petroleum jelly to the inside of the nostrils with a cotton swab to prevent drying.

4 If the air in your child's bedroom is dry, using a cool-mist vaporizer may help prevent nosebleeds from recurring.

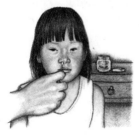

Description: A foreign object lodged in a nostril, possibly causing bleeding or discharge.

What you need to know:	When to get help:
• Small children often put foreign objects in their nose.	• Take your child to an emergency facility if you cannot *easily* remove the object from your child's nose.

Signs and symptoms:
• bleeding
• difficulty breathing
• a visible foreign object in the nose
• foul-smelling discharge from the nostrils (especially from one nostril)

Treatment:
• *If the object is visible and easy to grasp,* try to remove it with your fingers or round-ended tweezers.
• If the object cannot be removed, have your child blow his nose if he is able to do so.

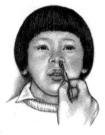

Caution:
• Do not try to remove an object that is not visible and easy to grasp; doing so may push the object farther into the nose and/or damage tissue.

Description: Injury to the nose causing bleeding, swelling, disfigurement, or impaired breathing.

What you need to know:	When to get help:
• Bruising under the eyes may occur after a day or two. • Very few nose injuries cause problems requiring immediate professional attention. The doctor may prefer to see your child after the swelling subsides.	• Call your doctor if: —Pain is severe or persists after treatment. —Bleeding cannot be controlled or recurs. —The nose seems misshapen. —Breathing through each nostril separately is difficult.

Signs and symptoms:
• swelling
• redness
• pain
• bleeding

Treatment:

1 Calm and reassure your child. Bleeding and swelling will be less severe if she relaxes.

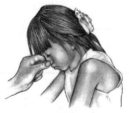

2 Stop bleeding as you would for a nosebleed.

3 Apply cold compresses to the nose to reduce swelling.

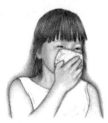

4 Give your child pain-relieving tablets or liquids (acetaminophen or ibuprofen), if needed. Follow the dosage recommended on the package label.

Description: Infection of the earlobe associated with pierced earrings or the piercing procedure.

What you need to know:	When to get help:
• Infections can result from posts that are too short, sensitivity to metals, improper piercing procedures, or improper care after piercing. Earrings should be made of good-quality metals (gold, silver, stainless steel), and the clasp should not be excessively tight or pinch the ear. • Never try to pierce your child's ears yourself.	• Call your doctor if: —Infection is severe. —Home treatment does not improve the condition in a few days. —Eczema develops (See page 108.)

Signs and symptoms:
• swelling/tenderness/redness of area around hole
• rawness and discharge; discharge dries and forms itchy crusting
• lumps in earlobes

Treatment:
• Remove earrings until infection clears up. The hole may close in the healing process, requiring repiercing.
• Clean front and back of lobe twice daily with alcohol, and apply antibiotic ointment.
• Follow the proper procedures for caring for newly pierced ears:
   —Insert only post earrings and don't remove for 4–6 weeks.
   —Clean front and back of the lobe twice daily with alcohol, and turn earrings several times daily.

Description: Inflammation of the white of the eyes and/or inner, lower lids.

What you need to know:	**When to get help:**
• Pinkeye is a common but rarely serious infection.	• Call your doctor if:
• Eye infections last about a week and may be contagious.	—You note redness, mattering, or discharge, especially if associated with fever over 102.5°F or swelling around the eye. Explain the symptoms in as much detail as possible. Your doctor may want to see your child or may prescribe medication over the phone.
• Not all "red eyes" are caused by bacteria or viruses; other causes include allergies and foreign objects in the eye.	
• Newborns with red eyes, tearing, and/or discharge may have a blocked tear duct.	—There is no improvement in 4–5 days with prescribed treatment.

Signs and symptoms:
• redness
• yellow-green discharge or mattering
• swollen eyelids
• increased tearing
• pain

Treatment:
• Apply warm compresses to reduce discomfort and to wipe away discharge.
• Have family members wash their hands carefully.
• Do not share your child's towels or washcloths with other family members.
• Administer antibiotic drops or ointment if prescribed by your doctor; do not use leftover eye medicines.

Description: Infestation of the intestine caused by a small parasite.

What you need to know:	When to get help:
• It is unlikely that pinworms cause abdominal pain, sleep disorders, or behavior problems. • Pinworm infections are not serious. They are common, easy to treat, and usually cause no symptoms. • Reinfestation is common because of transfer of the eggs from the rectal area to the mouth. • If you suspect pinworms, examine your child's rectal area with a flashlight 1–2 hours after he is asleep; pinworms are white and thread-like.	• Call your doctor if you suspect your child has pinworms.

Signs and symptoms:
• itching around the anus, especially at night
• vaginal irritation

Treatment:
• Administer medication prescribed by your health care professional for the child and other family members.
• Launder towels, bedding, clothes, and other items that come in contact with the infected child.

Description: A rash characterized by "salmon-colored" scaly, round, or oval lesions.

What you need to know:	When to get help:
• The rash will resolve itself without treatment in 4–6 weeks. • The rash may be preceded by a single patch, often on the trunk (herald patch). • The condition is asymptomatic (except for occasional itching).	• Call your doctor to diagnose the cause of the problem.

Signs and symptoms:
• rash, generally on the trunk
• minimal itching

Treatment:
• None, or mild hydrocortisone cream for itching.

Description: Infection of the lungs.

What you need to know:	**When to get help:**
• Pneumonia has multiple causes—usually viruses or bacteria. • It is rarely serious and is usually treated with antibiotics. • Some, but not all, pneumonias are contagious.	• Call your doctor if you suspect your child has pneumonia (especially if your child's cold is associated with labored breathing).

Signs and symptoms:
- fever
- cough
- labored breathing
- chest pains

Treatment:

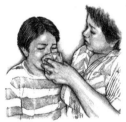

- Administer medications as prescribed by your doctor (frequently an antibiotic).
- Increase fluids.
- Give acetaminophen or ibuprofen for fever.

Related topics: Asthma; Cough; Cystic Fibrosis; Influenza ("Flu")

Description: An itchy rash caused by contact with poison ivy plants.

What you need to know:	**When to get help:**
• Poison ivy rash is not contagious and cannot be transferred to another person. • Poison ivy is a green, three-leafed plant that turns red in the fall. • The rash heals in about 2–3 weeks.	• Call your doctor if: —The rash requires identification. —Poison ivy is not effectively treated with home measures.

Signs and symptoms:
• red, itchy rash with small blisters
• often a straight-line rash with small blisters
• oozing from blisters

Treatment:
• Wash area immediately after contact with poison ivy plant; this will prevent further spread.
• Keep fingernails short.
• Apply cold compresses to affected area.
• Apply cortisone cream to relieve itching.
• Give your child antihistamines and/or oral cortisone prescribed by your doctor, especially if the rash is extensive.

Related topics: Allergy; Blister; Hives

Description: Ingestion of medicine, cleaning products, petroleum-based products, or other harmful substances.

What you need to know:	**When to get help:**
• Poisoning can be serious, but frequently can be managed at home. Prompt determination of the substance ingested and immediate treatment are essential. • Medicines, cleaning fluids, and houseplants are common causes of poisoning. • If possible, bring samples of the ingested substance and/or the vomitus with you to the hospital for analysis.	• Call your local emergency number (911) if your child is unconscious and/or has difficulty breathing. *Otherwise* • Call your local or regional Poison Control Center, doctor, or hospital immediately for instructions.

Signs and symptoms:
• sudden onset of illness or change in behavior, which may take many forms, depending on the substance ingested (Some possible symptoms are abdominal pain, diarrhea, blackouts, blurred vision, convulsions, choking, nausea, dizziness, confusion, and drowsiness.)

Treatment:
• If your child is conscious, try to determine what she swallowed.
• If instructions from the Poison Control Center, doctor, or hospital are not available, and your child has not swallowed a caustic substance (i.e., drain cleaner, disinfectant), or a petroleum product (i.e., gasoline or lighter fluid), give her 1 tablespoon (15 ml) of syrup of ipecac followed by 2 glasses of water to induce vomiting.
• For any swallowed liquid (not pills), give your child 2–3 glasses of water to dilute the liquid.

Caution:
• Do *not* induce vomiting if your child has swallowed a caustic substance, such as drain cleaner or disinfectant, or a petroleum product, such as gasoline or lighter fluid.

Related topics: Breathing Emergency; Convulsion; "Stomach Pain" (Abdominal Pain); Vomiting

Description: A viral infection of the spinal cord.

What you need to know:	**When to get help:**
• Polio is rare today because of universal immunization. • Immunizations are given at ages 2 months, 4 months, 15 months, and 5 years. • Immunizations are given orally or, in some cases, intramuscularly. • Most children who contract polio have no symptoms and will become immune.	• Call your doctor if your child is not immunized, is exposed to polio, or has the below signs and symptoms.

Signs and symptoms:
• fever
• muscle aches and pains
• stiff neck
• vomiting
• poor muscle function (paralysis)

Treatment:
• There is no specific treatment.

Description: Common red rash affecting 50 percent of newborn babies.

What you need to know:	When to get help:
• The rash is not serious and requires no treatment. • It will often last 4–16 days.	• Call your doctor if you need help to identify the rash.

Signs and symptoms:
• raised, red rash, frequently with pimples, on the face, trunk, and extremities

Treatment:
• None.

Description: Serious neurological disease frequently occurring after chicken pox or influenza, especially if aspirin is used in treatment.

What you need to know:	When to get help:
• The incidence of Reye's syndrome has practically disappeared since the discontinuation of aspirin for treatment of fever in children. • Do not give your child aspirin for treatment of fever, especially if he has chicken pox or flu.	• Call your doctor if you suspect your child has Reye's syndrome based on the below signs and symptoms.

Signs and symptoms:
• vomiting
• headache
• lethargy
• confusion
• poor coordination

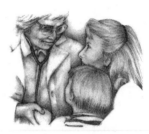

Treatment:
• None.

Related topics: Chicken Pox; Influenza ("Flu"); Vomiting

Description: An inflammation of the heart (valves and muscle) occurring as a rare complication of a strep throat.

What you need to know:	**When to get help:**
• Inadequately treated or undetected strep throat frequently precedes the development of rheumatic fever.	• Call your doctor if:
	—You need to discuss diagnosis and treatment of your child's sore throat.
• Only a small percentage of cases of untreated strep throats will develop rheumatic fever (less than 3 percent).	—Your child exhibits any of the below signs and symptoms suggesting rheumatic fever.
• All documented strep throats should be treated for a minimum of 10 days; do not discontinue antibiotics when your child feels well (usually after 24–48 hours).	
• There is no diagnostic test for rheumatic fever; diagnosis is made by the constellation of clinical findings.	

Signs and symptoms:
• fever
• rash
• arthritis (swollen, painful joints)
• heart murmur, chest pain
• unusual contortions or movements of the trunk or extremities *(chorea)*

Treatment:
• Prevention (adequate treatment of strep infection) is the best form of treatment.
• There is no home treatment.

Related topics: Arthritis; Sore Throat (Pharyngitis, "Strep Throat")

Description: Superficial skin infection caused by a fungus (not a worm).

What you need to know:	When to get help:
• Ringworm spreads by contact with an infected person or contaminated objects (combs, brushes, towels, and so on). • The rash may last approximately 6 weeks, but improvement with treatment should be noted in 1–2 weeks.	• Call your doctor if: —Diagnosis is unclear. —Ringworm is present on the scalp.

Signs and symptoms:

• pink, red, circular lesion with raised border and central clearing, which occurs on the face, trunk, extremities, groin (jock itch), or scalp (*tinea capitis*)

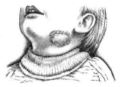

• patchy hair loss may be associated with scalp ringworm

Treatment:

• Administer oral medications for 4–6 weeks, as prescribed by your doctor for treatment of scalp ringworm.
• Use Tinactin or Lotrimin cream (over-the-counter) for ringworm infections not involving the scalp. Your doctor may prescribe a different cream.

Related topics: Athlete's Foot

Description: A potentially serious infection transmitted by a specific type of tick.

What you need to know:

- Rocky Mountain Spotted Fever is most prevalent on the Atlantic seaboard, but can occur in any part of the United States.
- It was first recognized in the Rocky Mountain states, thus its name.
- The earlier the diagnosis, the better the prognosis.
- Antibiotics will cure the disease if treated early (first 3 or 4 days).

When to get help:

- Call your doctor if:
  —You suspect your child has Rocky Mountain Fever based on the below signs and symptoms.
  —You are unable to remove the tick.

Signs and symptoms:

- fever
- headache
- chills
- muscle aches
- rash beginning on wrist, palms, ankles, and soles, which spreads centrally

Treatment:

- Use insect repellents, protective clothing, and always inspect your child for ticks, especially if you live in a wooded area.
- Remove attached ticks carefully. (See Lyme Disease, page 149, for tick removal.)
- Administer medication as prescribed by your doctor.

Description: A viral infection in infants and young children characterized by fever, rash, and, possibly, respiratory or gastrointestinal symptoms.

What you need to know:	**When to get help:**
• Roseola is caused by a specific virus (Human Herpesvirus 6) related to, but different from, other herpes viruses. • There is no treatment or prevention, and the disease is usually very mild. • It is most common in children ages 3–12 months. • A convulsion may occur at the outset of the illness, but it is rarely serious. • A rash may or may not develop after 3–5 days of fever.	• Call your doctor if you are concerned about the cause of fever, or if the diagnosis is unclear before the rash develops. • Call your local emergency number (911) if your child's seizure lasts more than 5 minutes.

Signs and symptoms:
• fever (often 103–105°F) lasting 3–5 days
• rash develops after fever resolves
• cold symptoms, vomiting, diarrhea in some infants

Treatment:
• Give your child acetaminophen or ibuprofen for fever. (See dosage charts, pages 19–21.)
• Treat convulsions. (See Convulsion, page 89.)

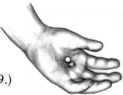

Description: Mite infestation of the skin, characterized by very itchy lesions.

What you need to know:	When to get help:
• Scabies is much more irritating than serious. • Scabies needs close, prolonged contact to spread; therefore, it is often spread at school. • Multiple family members are often affected.	• Call your doctor if you suspect your child has scabies.

Signs and symptoms:
• red, itchy bumps commonly located on wrists, creases of elbow, armpits, and webbing between fingers and toes

Treatment:
• Give your child cool baths or compresses.
• Apply special ointment or lotion as prescribed by your doctor.
• Check all family members for symptoms, and treat with prescribed medication.
• Launder all clothing, bedding, and towels in hot water.

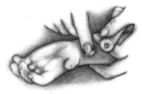

Description: Strep throat infection with a red rash.

What you need to know:	**When to get help:**
• Scarlet fever is merely strep throat with a rash, and it is no more serious than ordinary strep throat. • Scarlet fever is easily treated with antibiotics.	• Call your doctor for diagnostic confirmation of sore throat and rash.

Signs and symptoms:
- fever
- headache
- sore throat
- swollen neck glands
- sandpaper-like rash on face and body

Treatment:
- Give acetaminophen or ibuprofen.
- Offer throat soothers (lozenges, cold liquids).
- Administer antibiotics for 10 days; don't stop until you use up all the medicine, even if your child feels better after a few days.

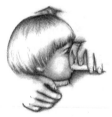

Related topics: Sore Throat (Pharyngitis, "Strep Throat"); Tonsillitis

Description: A curvature of the vertebral column (spine).

What you need to know:	**When to get help:**
• Scoliosis is most common in prepubescent girls, especially during periods of rapid growth. • Your health care professional will perform a special exam to detect this problem. • If detected early or if mild, surgery may be avoided.	• Call your doctor if you suspect scoliosis; prompt evaluation by your physician may prevent surgery.

Signs and symptoms:
• often none, especially with mild or moderate curvatures
• one shoulder or hip may appear higher than the other

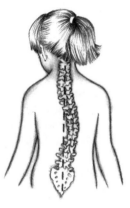

Treatment:
• Use bracing if recommended by a bone specialist.
• Surgery in some cases.

Description: Viral infection characterized by a specific rash caused by reemergence of the chicken pox virus.

What you need to know:	When to get help:
• Shingles is caused by the same virus that causes chicken pox. • It is very uncommon in children under age 10. • It generally resolves in 1–2 weeks. • Shingles tends to be more painful in adults than children. • If it occurs in children, it often does so in those who developed chicken pox before they were 1 year old and, therefore, did not develop complete immunity.	• Call your doctor for identification of the rash.

Signs and symptoms:
• grouped blisters, which are occasionally painful
• rash that tends to follow the nerve lines of the body

Treatment:
• There is no specific treatment for shingles.
• Apply wet compresses.
• Give acetaminophen or ibuprofen if the condition is painful.

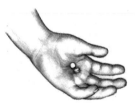

Related topics: Chicken Pox

Description: A dangerous decrease in vital bodily functions.

What you need to know:	**When to get help:**
• Shock may result from injuries with extensive blood loss, a severe allergic reaction, a serious infection, intense pain, extreme fear, or heart failure. • If shock results from blood loss, stop the bleeding before treating the shock.	• Call your local emergency number (911) if you suspect shock. Shock requires immediate treatment to prevent damage to vital organs and tissues.

Signs and symptoms:
• pale, cool, clammy skin
• dizziness/faintness
• thirst
• nausea/vomiting
• rapid, shallow breathing
• weak, rapid pulse

Treatment:

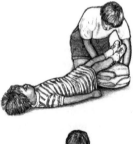

• If your child is conscious and *doesn't* have a head or chest injury with difficulty breathing, place her on her back and elevate her feet 8–12 inches.
• If your child is conscious and has a head or chest injury or difficulty breathing, elevate her head, but not her feet.
• Cover your child with a blanket or jacket to keep her warm.

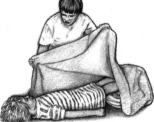

Description: A sudden, unexplained death of an infant (under age 12 months) in which the history or autopsy fails to reveal the cause of death.

What you need to know:	When to get help:
• Peak incidence of SIDS occurs in children ages 2–4 months. • The incidence of SIDS is higher in the winter months, in premature infants, and in lower socioeconomic groups. • Most deaths attributed to SIDS occur when infants are sleeping. • The cause of SIDS is unknown, but it is probably related to immaturity of the heart and breathing controls.	• Call your local emergency number (911) if your child is not breathing. Attempt CPR. (See Breathing Emergency—For Infants under 1 Year, page 53.)

Treatment:
• Place your infant on his back to sleep—this practice has significantly reduced the incidence of SIDS.
• For more information about SIDS, and to obtain counseling and contact with other parents, contact the SIDS Alliance, 1314 Bedford Avenue, Suite 210, Baltimore, MD 21208, (800) 221-7437. Phone lines are open Monday through Friday from 9 A.M. to 5 P.M., Eastern standard time. In case of an emergency, you will be connected to a counselor 24 hours a day.

Description: Inflammation of the lining of the sinuses.

What you need to know:	**When to get help:**
• Green nasal discharge is common with colds and generally resolves in 7–8 days.	• Call your doctor if your child's cold lasts more than 10 days and is accompanied by green nasal discharge, cough, and/or sinus pain.
• X-ray may occasionally be helpful in diagnosing sinusitis; however, there is no good test to verify the diagnosis.	
• Sinusitis is treated with antibiotics.	
• Diagnosis should be considered if your child's cold symptoms persist longer than 10 days and are associated with the below signs and symptoms.	

Signs and symptoms:
• cold, with or without greenish nasal discharge, lasting longer than 10 days
• pain over the sinuses
• fever
• cough (day and night)

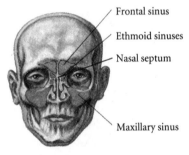

Frontal sinus

Ethmoid sinuses

Nasal septum

Maxillary sinus

Treatment:
• Administer medications as prescribed by your physician; these may include decongestants, nasal drops or spray, and/or antibiotics.

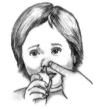

Related topics: Cold; Headaches

Description: An irritation of the throat or tonsils frequently caused by bacteria or viruses.

What you need to know:
- Sore throats are caused, most often, by minor irritations or viruses.
- Most children with colds complain of sore throats, especially upon awakening, which may not require a visit to your doctor.
- Children with colds and coughs accompanied by sore throat are highly unlikely to have strep throat; therefore, a throat swab for strep or antibiotics are not indicated.
- Your doctor should do a strep test before treating your child with antibiotics.
- If strep throat is diagnosed, continue antibiotics for 10 full days.
- Strep throats are less common in children under age 5 or 6 or during the summer months.

When to get help:
- Call your doctor if your child's sore throat is associated with a fever over 102°F or is not accompanied by cold symptoms.

Signs and symptoms:
- throat pain
- pain with swallowing
- swollen lymph glands in neck
- "white spots" noted on red enlarged tonsils

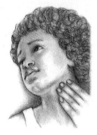

Treatment:
- Give acetaminophen or ibuprofen for pain and fever.
- Offer lozenges, soothing liquids.
- Administer antibiotics after the diagnosis of strep throat is confirmed.

Related topics: Diphtheria; Mononucleosis ("Mono"); Tonsillitis

Description: A foreign object embedded in the outer layer of skin.

What you need to know:	When to get help:
• Many splinters can be removed at home. • It is important to remove the entire splinter to avoid infection. • If the splinter is not easily grasped, soaking the affected area in warm water may help bring the object to the surface.	• Call your doctor if: —The splinter is deeply embedded and you cannot grasp the end. —Signs of infection develop (increasing redness, swelling, pain).

Treatment:

1 If the splinter is visible, grasp its end with tweezers, and pull it out.

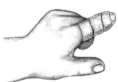

2 Free an embedded splinter with a needle cleaned with alcohol. Make a small hole over the head of the splinter; lift the end until you can grasp it with a tweezers and pull it out.

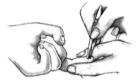

3 Wash the area with soap and water after splinter removal.

4 Leave the area exposed to air or apply a bandage.

Related topics: Cuts, Wounds, Scrapes; Tetanus ("Lock Jaw")

Description: A *sprain* is the tearing and/or stretching of a ligament; a *strain* is the tearing and/or stretching of muscle fibers or tendons ("pulled muscle").

What you need to know:	When to get help:
• Most muscle strains are minor and respond to symptomatic treatment and 1–2 days of limited activity.	• Call your doctor if:
• Sprains are relatively uncommon in younger children.	—The pain or swelling is severe.
• If you suspect a fracture, see Broken Bone (Fracture).	—Your child's ability to move the affected area is limited.
• Basic treatment principles for a sprain or a strain are Rest, Ice, Compression, Elevation (RICE).	—A bone is deformed and possibly broken.
	—The injured area remains painful, or your child is unable to apply pressure to the injured area after 48 hours of home treatment.

Signs and symptoms:
• pain, tenderness
• swelling
• cramping or stiffness
• limitation of joint mobility
• bruising

Treatment:

1 Have your child *rest* in a comfortable position.

2 Apply an *ice* pack to the injured area for 10–15 minutes to reduce swelling and pain. If swelling persists, reapply the cold compress, pausing every 15–20 minutes, until the swelling decreases.

3 If your child has an injury to the leg, ankle, or knee, apply an elastic bandage *(compression)* to the affected area firmly, but not tightly.

4 If possible, *elevate* the injured area above heart level to slow blood flow and reduce swelling.

5 Give your child pain-relieving tablets or liquids (acetaminophen or ibuprofen), if needed. Follow the dosage recommended on the package label.

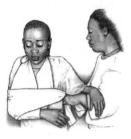

6 If your child has an injury to the shoulder, elbow, or wrist, immobilize the arm with a triangular cloth sling, and tie the sling to the body. (See Treatments and Procedures: Slings, page 25.)

7 After 48 hours, if pain and swelling have decreased, have your child try to move the affected joint in all directions.

8 Keep pressure off the injured area until the pain subsides. Your child can return to normal function as soon as she is able. However, avoid vigorous activity for approximately 2 weeks.

Related topics: Broken Bone (Fracture)

Description: Pain in the abdominal area.

What you need to know:	When to get help:
• There are many causes of abdominal pain, most of which are not serious and can be managed at home. • The associated symptoms (*e.g.,* vomiting, diarrhea) are important in determining the diagnosis. • Very sudden onset of pain in a well child is usually not serious and can be observed before calling a physician.	• Call your doctor if: —Pain persists longer than 3–4 hours. —The associated symptoms (fever, vomiting, diarrhea) are a concern. —Your child seems quite ill from the pain.

Signs and symptoms:
• localized or generalized pain, which may or may not be accompanied by fever, vomiting, or diarrhea

Treatment:
• Apply heating pads to abdomen.
• Offer clear liquids, if desired.
• Observe for persistent pain or associated symptoms.

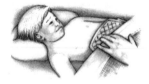

Related topics: Appendicitis; Constipation; Diarrhea; Vomiting

Description: Noncontagious infection of the glands located in the eyelids.

What you need to know:	When to get help:

• Many sties can be treated at home and are not serious.	• Call your doctor if:
	  —The sty does not improve in 3 days.
	  —If the eyelid or area around the eye becomes red or swollen.

Signs and symptoms:
• redness, swelling of the lid margin
• "pimple" on the lid margin

Treatment:
• Apply a wet compress for 10–15 minutes, 4–6 times a day.
• Do not probe, rub, or squeeze the sty.

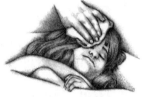

Related topics: Pink Eye (Conjunctivitis)

Description: Usually a first-degree burn involving the outer layer of skin, however it may be more severe. (See also, Burn.)

What you need to know:	When to get help:
• Sunburns are uncomfortable, but are usually not serious—except occasionally in small infants. • Repeated sunburns can increase the risk of skin cancer. • Prevention is the best form of treatment. • Infants should not be exposed to intense sun.	• Call your doctor if sunburn: —Causes headache or if pain is uncontrollable. —Is associated with blistering. —Is associated with symptoms of dehydration (light-headedness, dry mouth, decreased urine output).

Signs and symptoms:
• redness
• tenderness and/or pain
• possible blistering (with more serious forms)

Treatment:
• Take preventative measures:
—Use a sunscreen with an SPF of at least 15 for adults or SPF 30 (or sunblock) for infants and small children.
—Limit sun exposure in small infants.
—Have your child wear a hat with a broad brim to shade the face.
—Avoid the sun between the hours of 11 A.M. and 2 P.M.
• Give cool baths or apply cold compresses.
• Offer acetaminophen and ibuprofen for pain.
• Apply ointments or sprays as prescribed by your doctor.

Related topics: Blister; Burn

Description: The swallowing of a nondissolving object.

What you need to know:	When to get help:
• Most objects (80–90 percent) pass through the intestinal tract without causing problems. • Coins are the most common objects ingested. • Once objects are in the stomach, more than 95 percent will pass without difficulty. • Sharp, irregular objects are more prone to becoming lodged than smooth ones. • Most objects will pass in 3–4 days, but some may take as long as 4–6 weeks.	• Call your doctor if: —Your child complains of chest pain and difficulty swallowing. —The swallowed object is sharp or irregular (e.g., an open safety pin).

Signs and symptoms:
• often none, other than older children's reports that an object was swallowed (In younger children, disappearance of the object is the only sign.)

Treatment:
• Observe the child's stools for appearance of the object.
• Your doctor may do an X-ray to follow the progress of the swallowed object; in certain cases, a specialist will remove the object.

Related topics: Breathing Emergency; Choking; Cough

Description: An inflammation (infection) in the ear canal, common in swimmers.

What you need to know:
• Frequent or sustained exposure of the ear canal to water reduces its protection against infection.
• It is important to dry ears after swimming and showering.
• Do not attempt to dry ears with cotton swabs; these may cause ittitation and increase the risk of infection.

When to get help:
• Call your doctor if your child has the below signs and symptoms.

Signs and symptoms:
• pain, especially when pulling on the ear or pressing on the front part of the ear
• discharge
• swollen ear canal
• itching
• decreased hearing

Treatment:
• Dry ears after showering and swimming by shaking out the water, drying with corner of towel or tissue, or using a hair dryer at low setting held a few inches from the ear.
• Use a solution before and after swimming, as recommended by your doctor, for prevention.
• Administer special antibiotic drops as prescribed by your doctor.

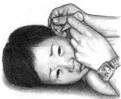

Related topics: Ear Infections

Description: Enlargement of the lymph glands, usually noted on the neck (front or back), or occasionally in the armpits or groin.

What you need to know:	When to get help:
• It is common to feel small lymph glands in your child's neck (less than 1 cm. in diameter).	• Call your doctor if your child's lymph glands are red and painful and there is associated fever.
• Lymph glands contain special cells that help the body combat and contain infection.	
• Lymph glands act as filters and prevent germs from invading the bloodstream.	
• Swelling indicates that the glands are doing their job.	
• When the glands themselves become infected (red, swollen), they may require treatment with antibiotics.	

Signs and symptoms:
• tender, occasionally red, swollen glands
• possible fever

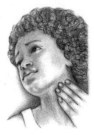

Treatment:
• Usually none unless signs of infection develop.
• Administer antibiotics as prescribed for infection.

Related topics: Mononucleosis ("Mono"); Sore Throat (Pharyngitis, "Strep Throat"); Tonsillitis

Description: Discomfort sometimes noted during the eruption of teeth.

What you need to know:	When to get help:
• Teeth erupt for 3–4 years; thus, every behavior problem or other symptom should not be attributed to teething. • Colds, fever, diarrhea, and constipation are usually not symptoms of teething.	• Call your doctor if you have concerns about symptoms associated with teething.

Signs and symptoms:
• drooling
• irritability
• chewing fingers or other objects

Treatment:
• Rub your child's gums with your finger.
• Offer rubber teething rings. (Teething rings kept in the freezer are too hard.)
• Avoid medications that are rubbed on gums; they are not helpful since they wash out of the mouth very quickly.

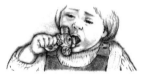

Description: Testes that do not descend permanently into scrotum and remain in the abdomen or groin.

What you need to know:	When to get help:
• Testes usually migrate into the scrotum before birth; in some cases, the testes may complete their descent shortly after birth. • Testes that are undescended are at increased risk for twisting, becoming injured, or developing cancer. • Occasionally, testes are retractile (slip into and out of the scrotum). • Surgery before 1 year of age is indicated to preserve testicular function.	• Call your doctor if you suspect your child has an undescended testicle.

Signs and symptoms:
• testicles not present in the scrotum
• scrotum may appear unusually small

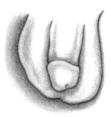

Treatment:
• Surgery, if the testes are undescended.
• Check for retractile testes by placing your child in a tub of warm water, which often causes the testes to descend into the scrotum. If you are unsure, have your doctor confirm the diagnosis.

Description: Twisting of the testes on its cord.

What you need to know:	**When to get help:**
• Although there are other causes of pain and swelling of the scrotum, immediate evaluation is imperative. • Immediate surgical intervention is necessary to treat torsion.	• Call your doctor if your child complains of pain and/or swelling in the scrotal area.

Signs and symptoms:
• intense pain in scrotum or groin
• nausea/vomiting
• swollen scrotum

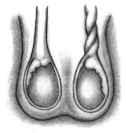

Treatment:
• Surgery.

Related topics: Hernia

Description: An infectious disease causing spasms of the muscles.

What you need to know:	**When to get help:**
• Tetanus is caused by a toxin produced by a bacteria (Clostridium tetani). • Tetanus occurs in a contaminated wound. • Disease can be prevented with regular tetanus immunization. (Required every 7 years after receiving the primary immunization in infancy.)	• Call your doctor if your child has a contaminated wound and her immunizations are incomplete.

Signs and symptoms:
• stiffness/spasms in jaw muscles
• difficulty swallowing
• stiff, rigid extremities
• difficulty breathing

Treatment:
• Prevention with immunization is the best form of treatment.
• Prompt, thorough cleaning of wounds is essential.

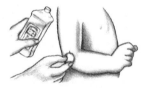

Related topics: Bites, Stings (Animal, Human, Snake); Cuts, Wounds, Scrapes

Description: A yeast infection of the tongue and mouth that occurs in infants.

What you need to know:	**When to get help:**
• White patches resemble milk curds, but are not easily removed when wiped with a cloth.	• Call your doctor if you suspect your child has thrush.

Signs and symptoms:
• white patches on the inside of cheeks, mouth, gums, and tongue

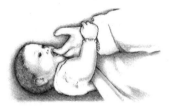

Treatment:
• Administer oral medication (Nystatin) as prescribed by your doctor.

Description: Brief, involuntary, repetitive movements of small muscle groups.

What you need to know:	**When to get help:**
• Simple tics are not uncommon, and the specific cause is usually not determined. • Stress may increase the frequency of tics. • Tics (simple) will often last up to 6–9 months and resolve without treatment.	• Call your doctor if: —Motor, muscle tics last more than 6–9 months. —Underlying stressors require counseling. —Motor (facial muscle twitching) and vocal tics (cough, throat clearing) coexist; this may indicate your child has Tourette's syndrome.

Signs and symptoms:
• facial muscle twitching
• frequent blinking
• coughing
• throat clearing

Treatment:
• Determine underlying stressors, if present.
• Ignore the tic, and it will resolve sooner.

Description: An inflammation (infection) of the tonsils most often caused by viruses or strep.

What you need to know:	When to get help:
• Tonsils contain lymph tissue, which aids the body in defense against infection. • Tonsils increase in size during childhood, and begin to decrease after age 6 or 7 years. • Tonsils frequently enlarge in children with common colds. They are not infected, but are helping to fight the infection. • There are very few reasons to remove tonsils; size alone usually is not a good reason. • If tonsils are infected, your child may need a strep test.	• Your child may require a strep test if the below signs and symptoms are present. • Call your doctor if drooling or difficulty swallowing develops. If this occurs with a high fever, it may indicate an abscess of the tonsils (usually in older children or adolescents.).

Signs and symptoms:
• sore throat
• swollen, inflamed tonsils, with or without white or yellow lesions

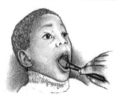

Treatment:
• Give your child acetaminophen or ibuprofen to reduce fever. (See dosage charts, pages 19–21.)
• Offer lozenges, soothing liquids.
• Treat cold symptoms, if present.
• Administer antibiotics, as prescribed by your doctor, if strep test is positive.

Related topics: Cold; Mononucleosis ("Mono"); Sore Throat (Pharyngitis, "Strep Throat")

Description: Pain in a specific tooth, usually caused by tooth decay or injury.

What you need to know:	When to get help:
• Tooth decay is largely preventable with proper brushing, flossing, and fluoride treatments.	• Call your dentist if you suspect your child has a toothache.
• Between ages 12 and 18 months, your child should visit the dentist to discuss oral hygiene.	
• Diagnosis of a toothache is not always obvious, i.e., unexplained facial pain or swelling may be caused by a tooth abscess.	

Signs and symptoms:
• pain, frequently worsened by cold or by tapping the tooth with a blunt object (Popsicle stick)
• gum area near the tooth is red, swollen, tender

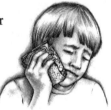

Treatment:
• Give acetaminophen or ibuprofen for pain relief. (See dosage charts, pages 19–21.)
• Apply ice packs to your child's jaw.

Description: A contagious disease caused by a bacteria that most commonly affects the lung, but any organ system can be involved.

What you need to know:	**When to get help:**
• TB is spread from respiratory secretions of patients with active TB. • Most often, your child will not have symptoms of TB, but a special skin test will indicate whether he has contracted the bacteria. • Incidence of TB has increased dramatically since the mid-1980s due to the increase in HIV infection (which makes one more susceptible to TB), immigration, and intravenous drug use. • TB may involve almost any organ in the body, but generally starts in the lung.	• Call your doctor if your child has been in contact with someone with active TB.

Signs and symptoms:
• may be none (common in children)
• persistent cough
• fever
• lack of energy (easily fatigued)
• weight loss, decreased appetite
• night sweats

Treatment:
• Drug treatment can cure TB.
• Treatment is required even if your child has only a positive skin test and no other symptoms.

Related topics: Cough; Pneumonia

Description: A localized erosion of the lining of the stomach or duodenum (first part of the small intestine).

What you need to know:	When to get help:
• Ulcers are much less common in children than in adults.	• Talk to your docot if you suspect your child has an ulcer.
• A child between the ages of 5 and 13 years who complains of recurrent midabdominal pain without other symptoms over a period of weeks or months usually does not have an ulcer.	• A specialist may have to look into the stomach with a special tube (endoscope) to make a diagnosis.
• The bacteria *Helicobacter pylori* is a treatable cause of ulcers.	

Signs and symptoms: *(vary with the age of the child):*
• recurrent pain in the upper abdomen
• vomiting blood (more common in infants)
• black bowel movements (indicates blood in stool)
• pain between meals or at night

Treatment:
• Administer medications as prescribed by your doctor.

Description: Discharge (occasionally blood-tinged) noted after the cord falls off.

What you need to know:	**When to get help:**
• Oozing or slight swelling of the cord stump is normal. • Persistent oozing and the presence of red, irritated skin is not normal and should be checked by a doctor.	• Call your doctor if: —Oozing persists despite using alcohol wipes. —Increasing redness or tenderness develops at the base of the cord (may indicate infection).

Signs and symptoms:
• moist oozing from cord
• small drops of blood in the discharge
• red skin around the cord base
• swollen umbilical cord *(umbilical cord granuloma)*

Treatment:
• Clean cord stump with alcohol wipes several times daily.
• Your doctor may apply a drying medicine (silver nitrate).
• Make sure the cord stump doesn't adhere to the diaper. You may need to apply Vaseline in addition to the ointment used by the doctor.

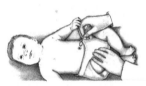

Description: An infection in the urinary system caused by bacteria.

What you need to know:	When to get help:
• Many urinary tract infections (UTIs) are caused by bacteria from the child's body (intestinal tract) that travel up the urethra (tube from bladder) and infect the urinary system. • The diagnosis is made by taking a sample of urine (sterile), examining it under a microscope (urinalysis), and doing a culture to identify the causative bacteria. • UTIs occur with increased frequency in uncircumcised, as compared with circumcised, male infants (9 to 1).	• Call your doctor if signs or symptoms of urinary tract infection develop. • If your child has a urinary tract infection, special diagnostic tests will be performed—kidney ultrasound, X-ray exam of voiding (VCUG).

Signs and symptoms:
• burning or pain on urination
• frequent urination
• discolored urine with a strong odor
• fever
• abdominal or back pain
• vomiting
• bedwetting in a child previously dry

Treatment:
• Administer antibiotics as prescribed by your doctor.
• Increase fluid intake.
• Take preventive measures:
  —Avoid bubble baths.
  —Teach girls to wipe from front to back.
  —Have girls wear cotton underpants.

Related topics: Bedwetting

Description: A short- or long-term vision impairment.

What you need to know:	When to get help:

• Vision problems most often occur during middle childhood (school age).
 • Nearsightedness (myopia), or the inability to see distant objects, is the most common problem.
 • Farsightedness (hyperopia) is the inability to see objects that are close.
 • Both types of vision problems may require glasses.
	• Call your doctor or an eye care specialist if:
	   —Your child develops the sudden onset of crossed eyes.
	   —The below signs or symptoms are present.
	   —You suspect your child may have a vision problem because of your family history.

Signs and symptoms:
• head tilting
• crossed eyes
• looking out corner of eyes, squinting
• eye rubbing
• sitting close to TV
• holding objects close to examine

Treatment:
• Varies with the problem, as diagnosed by your eye care specialist.

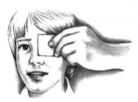

Description: Forceful regurgitation of food or fluid due to variety of conditions.

What you need to know:	When to get help:
• Many infants "spit up" and occasionally vomit. The condition is usually not serious unless associated with poor weight gain or excessive coughing. • Vomiting is one of the body's defenses to rid itself of infection or toxin. It is potentially serious if persistent or if it recurs frequently—either can lead to dehydration. • A viral infection of the stomach and/or intestines (gastroenteritis) is the most common cause of vomiting.	• Call your doctor if: —Your child's vomiting lasts more than 6 hours. —The vomiting is accompanied by abdominal pain, fever, or headache.

Treatment:
• Give nothing by mouth until vomiting has subsided for 1½ to 2 hours. Then, give small amounts of preferred liquids (1 teaspoon to 1 tablespoon every 10–15 minutes), increasing gradually as tolerated.
• Do not use over-th-counter vomiting medications.

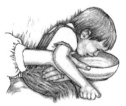

Related topics: Diarrhea; Encephalitis; Gastroenteritis; Meningitis; Reye's Syndrome

Description: Skin growth caused by specific viruses.

What you need to know:	**When to get help:**
• The majority of warts will resolve without treatment over an extended period of time (up to 2–3 years). • Except when present on feet, warts rarely cause symptoms. • Warts often recur even after treatment.	• Call your doctor if the wart is causing symptoms or is cosmetically unacceptable.

Signs and symptoms:
• raised, rough growth found anywhere on the body

Treatment:
• Most warts do not require treatment unless they are causing symptoms (bleeding, pain), or if the child is constantly picking at the wart.
• Try over-the-counter treatments, especially those with salicylic acid.
• Use the treatment recommended by your doctor; the specific treatment depends on the size of the wart.

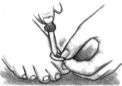

Description: A highly contagious bacterial disease characterized by a paroxysmal cough.

What you need to know:	**When to get help:**
• Most children who contract this disease do not have a "whoop" (defined below). • Some adults acquire whooping cough because they have diminished immunity to this disease. These adults usually have a mild form of the disease, with a persistent cough being the only symptom, and so they are frequently not diagnosed or treated. They may transmit this infection to infants. • Pertussis is most serious in very young infants. • DPT (diphtheria, pertussis, tetanus) immunizations at ages 2 months, 4 months, and 6 months will prevent most cases. • A new pertussis vaccine *(Acellular Pertussis)* has fewer side effects than the old vaccine.	• Call your doctor if: —Your infant or child is incompletely immunized and has been exposed to whooping cough. —A cough lasts longer than 2 weeks.

Signs and symptoms:
• coughing paroxysms ending in a prolonged high-pitched crowing sound (whoop)
• cold symptoms lasting 10–14 days, without fever, preceding the coughing spasms
• vomiting

Treatment:
• Prevention by vaccination is the best form of treatment.
• Hospitalization with careful monitoring is required for young infants and some children with pertussis.
• Administer erythromycin, as prescribed by your doctor, to prevent spread of the disease to other family members. The antibiotic will not hasten recovery.

Related topics: Cough; Croup

PART FOUR

Appendix

Guide to Resources

Books

Pregnancy and Childbirth

Bard, Maureen. *Getting Organized for Your New Baby.* *(Meadowbrook)*

Carter, John Mack (ed.). *The Good Housekeeping Illustrated Book of Pregnancy and Baby Care.* (Hearst)

Eisenberg, Arlene, and Sandee Hathaway, et. al. *What to Expect When You're Expecting: The First Year.* (Workman Publishing)

Johnson, Robert V. (ed.). *Mayo Clinic Complete Book of Pregnancy and Baby's First Year.* (William Morrow & Co.)

Simkin, Penny, Janet Whalley, and Ann Keppler. *Pregnancy, Childbirth, and the Newborn.* (Meadowbrook)

Swinney, Bridget. *Eating Expectantly: A Practical and Tasty Guide to Prenatal Nutrition.* (Meadowbrook)

Child Development

Brazelton, T. Berry. *Touchpoints: The Essential Reference, Your Child's Emotional & Behavioral Development.* (Addison-Wesley)

Eisenberg, Arlene, et. al. *What to Expect When You're Expecting: Toddler Years.* (Workman Publishing)

Leach, Penelope. *Babyhood, Your Baby & Child From Birth to Age Five.* (Knopf)

Turecki, Stanley. *The Difficult Child.* (Bantam Books)

Weiss, Lynn. *How to Read Your Child Like a Book.* (Meadowbrook)

Parenting

Einzig, Mitchell. *Baby and Child Emergency First-Aid Handbook.* (Meadowbrook)

Ferber, Richard. *Solve Your Child's Sleep Problems.* (Simon & Schuster)

Gookin, Sandra Hardin, and Dan Gookin (ed.). *Parenting for Dummies.* (IDG Books)

Greydanus, Donald E. (ed.). *Caring for Your Adolescent Ages 12–21 Years.* (Bantam Books)

Jones, Sandy, with Werner Freitag and eds. of *Consumer Reports. Guide to Baby Products* (5th ed.). (Consumer Reports Books)

Kurcinka, Mary Sheedy. *Raising Your Spirited Child: A Guide for Parents Whose Child is More Intense, Sensitive, Perceptive, Persistent, Energetic.* (HarperPerennial)

Lansky, Vicki. *Feed Me! I'm Yours.* (Meadowbrook)

Lansky, Vicki. *Practical Parenting Tips* (Meadowbrook)

Lighter, Dawn. *Gentle Discipline.* (Meadowbrook)

Markel, Howard, and Frank A. Oski. *The Practical Pediatrician, The A-Z Guide to Your Child's Health, Behavior, and Safety.* (W.H. Freeman)

Schmitt, Barton D. *Your Child's Health: The Parent's Guide to Symptoms, Emergencies, Common Illnesses, Behavior, and School Problems.* (Bantam Books)

Schor, Edward L. (ed-in-chief). *Caring for Your School Age Child: Ages 5–12.* (Bantam Books)

Shelov, Steve (ed.). *Caring for Your Baby and Young Child Birth to Age 5 Years.* (American Academy of Pediatric Books)

Spock, Benjamin, and Michael Rothenberg. *Spock's New Baby and Child Care.* (Simon & Schuster)

Woolfson, Richard. *Child Care A to Z: The First Five Years.* (Meadowbrook)

Wyckoff, Jerry, and Barbara Unell. *Discipline without Shouting or Spanking: Practical Solutions to the Most Common Preschool Behavior Problems.* (Meadowbrook)

Magazines

American Baby, 249 West 17th Street, New York, NY 10011, (212) 645-0067. Written for expectant and new mothers, emphasizing health, nutrition, fashion, beauty tips, and more.

Baby Talk, 25 West 43rd Street, New York, NY 10036-7406, (212) 840-4200. Written for expectant and new mothers, focusing on the first year of life.

Child, 110 Fifth Avenue, New York, NY 10011-5699, (212) 463-1000. Written for parents of children aged up to 12, including articles on child development, behavior, health, nutrition, and education.

Mothering, P.O. Box 1690, Santa Fe, NM 87504, (505) 984-8116. Written for mothers, fathers, and health care workers, emphasizing self-care tips and ways of meeting and coping with the challenges of parenthood.

Parenting, 301 Howard Street, 17th Floor, San Francisco, CA 94105, (415) 546-7575. Written for the educated contemporary woman, emphasizing the demands of childrearing, personal growth, and family life.

Parents', 685 Third Avenue, New York, NY 10017-4052, (212) 878-8700. Written for young women aged 18–34 with growing children.

Working Mother, 230 Park Avenue, New York, NY 10169-0005, (212) 551-9500. Written for contemporary working women with children under age 18.

Resource Groups

American Academy of Pediatrics (AAP), 141 Northwest Point Boulevard, P.O. Box 927, Elk Grove Village, IL 60009-0927, Phone: (708) 228-5005, Fax: (708) 228-5097, e-mail: kidsdocs@aap.org. World Wide Web: http://www.aap.org. Professional medical society of pediatricians and pediatric subspecialists. Subdivisions include Accident and Poison Prevention; Early Childhood, Adoption, and Dependent Care; and Infectious Diseases. Operates a small member library of books and journals on pediatric medicine, office practice, and child health care policy. Publishes newsletters, journals, reports, guides, and handbooks.

American Red Cross National Headquarters (ARC), 431 18th Street NW, Washington, DC 20006, Phone: (202) 737-8300. Assists other Red Cross societies. Publishes booklets and an annual report.

Consumer Product Safety Commission, National Injury Information Clearinghouse, 5401 Westbard Avenue, Bethesda, MD 20207, Phone: (301) 504-0424, Toll-Free: (800) 638-CPSC, Fax: (301) 504-0025. Clearinghouse that collects and disseminates injury data and information on the causes and prevention of death, injury, and illness associated with consumer products and maintains detailed investigative reports of such injuries.

International Childbirth Education Association (ICEA), P.O. Box 20048, Minneapolis, MN 55420, Phone: (612) 854-8660, Toll-Free: (800) 624-4934 (for book orders only), Fax: (612) 854-8772, World Wide Web: http://www.icea.org. Purpose is to further the educational, physical, and emotional preparation of expectant parents for childbearing and breastfeeding. Offers a teacher certification program for childbirth educators. Publishes literature pertaining to family-centered maternity care, including journals and pamphlets. Operates a mail-order bookstore in Minneapolis, Minn., which makes available literature on all aspects of childbirth education and family-centered maternity care.

La Leche League International (LLLI), 1400 Meacham, Schaumburg, IL 60173, Phone: (708) 519-7730, Toll-Free: (800) LA-LECHE, Fax: (708) 519-0035, e-mail (to chat): lllol@library.ummed.edu, e-mail (to subscribe): listserv@ library.ummed.edu, World Wide Web: http://www.lalecheleague. org. Operates 550 breastfeeding resource centers in 48 countries. Promotes breastfeeding as an important element in the healthy development of the baby and mother, and as a means to encourage closer family relationships. Provides support through informal discussions and individualized counseling. Supplies information through publications, telephone service, and correspondence. Sponsors workshops, conferences, and seminars. Publishes booklets, journals, pamphlets, and books.

National Committee for the Prevention of Child Abuse (NCPCA), 332 South Michigan Avenue, Suite 1600, Chicago, IL 60604-4357, Phone: (312) 663-3520, Toll-Free: (800) CHILDREN, Fax: (312) 939-8962, e-mail: ncpca@childabuse.org. Seeks to stimulate greater public awareness of the influence, origins, nature, and effects of child abuse. Serves as a national advocate to prevent the neglect and physical, sexual, and emotional abuse of children. Conducts child abuse prevention programs. Publishes booklets, pamphlets, and journals.

National Information Center for Children and Youth with Disabilities (NICHCY), P.O. Box 1492, Washington, DC 20013, Phone: (202) 884-8200, Toll-Free: (800) 695-0285, Fax: (202) 884-8441, e-mail (to order publications list): gopher@aed.org, e-mail (to ask questions): nichcy@aed.org. Provides information to assist parents, educators, advocates, and others in helping children and youth with disabilities participate as fully as possible in school, at home, and in the community. Offers personal responses to specific questions. Gives referrals to other organizations and sources of help. Offers technical assistance to parents and professional groups. Publishes booklets, a free newsletter, papers, and informational packets.

National Institute of Mental Health (NIMH), 5600 Fishers Lane, Room 7-99, Rockville, MD 20857, Phone: (301) 443-3673, Fax: (301) 443-2578. Plans, conducts, fosters, and supports research, research training, and services on the brain, mental illness, and mental health, particularly the causes, prevention, diagnosis, and treatment of mental illness.

Parents Anonymous, 675 West Foothill Boulevard, Suite 220, Claremont, CA 91711-3416, Phone: (909) 621-6184, Fax: (909) 625-6304, e-mail: hn3831@handsnet.org. Works for the prevention and treatment of child abuse. Treatment blends support groups with self-help. Publishes a newsletter.

Parents without Partners, Inc. (PWP), 401 North Michigan Avenue, Chicago, IL 60611-4267, Phone: (312) 644-6610, Toll-Free: (800) 637-7974, Fax: (312) 321-6869. Researches single-parent topics. Promotes the study of and works to alleviate the problems of single parents (custodial and noncustodial) in relation to the welfare and upbringing of their children and the acceptance into the general social order of single parents and their children. Publishes brochures and manuals.

SIDS Alliance, 1314 Bedford Avenue, Suite 210, Baltimore, MD 21208, Phone: (410) 653-8226, Toll-Free: (800) 221-SIDS, Fax: (410) 653-8709. Serves as a central source of medical and scientific information about SIDS. Works to eliminate SIDS through research. Assists bereaved parents who have lost a child to SIDS. Works with families and professionals in caring for infants at risk due to cardiac and respiratory problems.

United States Consumer Product Safety Commission, Washington, DC 20207, Toll-Free: (800) 638-2772, Fax: (301) 504-0051, e-mail (for general information): gopher services:cpse.gov, e-mail (to report products): info:cpse.gov. Provides information on the safety and effectiveness of consumer products.

Glossary

Italicized words are also defined separately.

abdomen the area of the body just below the diaphragm, containing the stomach, intestines, and other organs.

abscess an infected area filled with pus and surrounded by *inflammation*.

acetaminophen a drug commonly used for fever and pain, provided in suspension, liquid, and tablet form.

acetone a fragrant liquid ketone found in abnormal quantities in the urine of diabetics.

acid burn a burn caused by an acid, such as battery acid.

alkali burn a burn caused by a base, such as sodium hydroxide (ingredient in drain and oven cleaners).

allergen a substance that causes an *allergic reaction*.

allergic reaction the body's response to a specific *allergen*, e.g., sneezing, hives.*

anelgesic a pain reliever.

antibacterial ointment an ointment that contains agents that combat the growth of bacteria.

antibiotic a drug that combats bacterial growth.

antihistamine a class of drugs that treats allergies.

antitoxin a substance produced by the body that neutralizes a specific toxin *(poison)*.

anus the opening at the end of the *rectum*.

bacterial infection an infection caused by a variety of microorganisms.

bronchioles the smallest air passages in the lungs.

cardiogram the printed results of the heart's rate and rhythm.

Cold/Hot Pack a commercial product that is capable of being heated or chilled for use as a *compress*.

coma unconsciousness.

compress a cloth or container used to apply heat or cold to the body.

conjunctivitis an inflammation of the membranes covering the whites of the eye.

CPR (cardiopulmonary resuscitation) a technique used to revive people who have had cessation of breathing and/or heart function.

DPT immunization a vaccination providing protection against Diphtheria,* Pertussis (whooping cough),* and Tetanus.*

Dramamine a common anti*nausea* drug.

elixir a sweetened mixture of alcohol and water, used as the base for many medicines.

enzyme a chemical in the body that assists in certain chemical reactions, such as the breakdown of food into nutrients.

epiglottis a flap of tissue at the opening of the trachea (windpipe) that closes it off when food or drink is swallowed.

Eustachian tubes the tubes extending from the middle ear to the throat.

febrile refers to fever* or a feverish condition.

febrile seizure uncontrolled movements of limbs or generalized shaking (convulsion*) caused by fever.*

flu a short name for influenza.*

fungus a family of germs that may cause infection, most often skin infections.

generic a word applied to drugs sold under a descriptive or chemical name rather than a brand name. Generic drugs usually cost less than brand-name drugs.

*See Step-by-Step Treatment entry.

genetic refers to tendencies or physical characteristics acquired by inheritance, through the genes. Susceptibility to some illnesses is related to a person's genetic inheritance.

germ a common term used instead of *virus*, bacteria, or *fungus*.

groin the part of the body where the thighs join the trunk; the site of the genital organs.

hemangioma a type of birthmark* caused by a cluster of small blood vessels under the skin.

hemoglobin the protein in the blood that carries oxygen to the tissue.

hereditary refers to the traits or characteristics passed along *genetic*ally.

herpes viruses a group of *viruses* causing specific diseases; i.e., Herpes simplex 1* causes cold sores.*

hydrocortisone cream or ointment containing a hormone (cortisone) that reduces *inflammation.*

immobilize to render a body part stationary; a splint, for example, secures a broken bone* in a fixed position.

immunization substances that prevent specific disease; i.e., DPT, Polio.

incubation refers to the time between exposure to a disease and the onset of *symptoms.*

inflammation a sign of infection or injury that results in redness, swelling, and pain. The -itis at the end of many disease names often means inflammation of; e.g., Bronchitis* is an inflammation of the bronchial tubes.

insulin a hormone secreted by the pancreas necessary for the body's cells to utilize glucose for energy.

jaundice* yellow-green skin and whites of the eyes. Common in newborns and a result of liver or blood diseases.

"jock itch" a skin infection of the *groin* caused by a *fungus.*

joint a moveable part where two bones join, e.g., knee, shoulder.

lesion an injury or wound.

lethargy a state of reduced activity and/or consciousness.

ligament a connecting tissue that unites bones at a *joint* or muscles to bones.

lymphangitis an *inflammation* of the lymph vessels ("blood poisoning"*).

lymph glands (nodes) special cells that act as filters to help the body combat infection. They can become tender and enlarged in the neck (front or back), or occasionally in the armpits or *groin.*

Lytren a solution of water, minerals, and sugar, used in the treatment of vomiting* and diarrhea.*

malady a general term for a disorder or illness.

malaise an overall sense of not feeling well.

metabolism the complex chemical processes by which cells utilize oxygen, break down food, build tissue, and discard waste.

nasal aspirator a squeeze-ball device for removing fluids from the nasal passages.

nausea the feeling that one may vomit.*

nurse practitioner a nurse with graduate training (usually one or two years beyond the nursing degree) who has skills in providing primary care (health supervision) and treating minor illness.

optometrist a specialist who performs eye examinations.

ophthalmologist a medical doctor who specializes in eye disease and performs surgery.

*See Step-by-Step Treatment entry.

paramedics personnel with various types of medical training, but without a medical degree.

Pedialyte a solution of water, minerals, and sugar used in the treatment of vomiting* and diarrhea.*

pedodontist a dentist who specializes in the treatment of children.

plantar wart a type of wart* that occurs on the bottom of the foot.

poison any substance that, if inhaled or swallowed, can produce adverse effects.

postnasal drip the drainage of mucus from the nasal passages into the throat.

preventive health care a variety of measures designed to prevent medical problems, e.g., health supervision visits, *immunizations.*

puberty the time at which adult sexual characteristics begin to develop in children.

rabies a viral infection acquired after being bitten by a rabid animal (dog, bat, etc.).

rectum the lower part of the lower intestine, ending at the anus.

retractile testicle a *testicle* that, having once been in its proper place in the scrotal sac (scrotum*), temporarily retracts into the lower abdomen.

salivary glands the saliva-secreting glands located in the area where the jaw meets the neck.

scrotum the external sac that contains the *testicles.*

seizure a convulsion* consisting of uncontrollable movements of the arms and legs.

silver nitrate a chemical compound occasionally applied to the eyes of newborns to protect them against specific eye infections.

spasm a sudden, involuntary contraction of a muscle or group of muscles.

sputum the mucus produced by coughing.*

staphylococcus a family of bacteria causing pus infection (staph infections).

symptom an indicator of malfunction of the body frequently caused by a disease process.

syrup of ipecac a drug that induces vomiting,* to be used as directed by a health care professional or *poison* control center.

tepid refers to lukewarm temperatures.

testicle one of the male reproductive organs that produces sperm and male hormones.

tonsillectomy an operation to remove the *tonsils.*

tonsils the lymphoid structures at the back of the throat that can combat infection, and occasionally become infected.

torso the trunk of the body.

tourniquet a device used to stop bleeding.

tumor a localized swelling or protuberance.

ulcer an open, inflamed lesion of the skin or other tissue, e.g., stomach ulcer.

umbilical cord the tube-like cord supplying nutrition that connects a fetus to the placenta.

venom a *poison* (toxin) secreted by an animal or insect.

virus a germ that must live inside body cells to multiply. Viruses do not respond to *antibiotic* treatment, and most are self-limited (resolve without treatment).

yeast infection an infection caused by a specific organism (monilia). Common examples are thrush,* certain diaper rashes,* and (in adolescent females) vaginal infections.

*See Step-by-Step Treatment entry.

Index

The **bolded** numbers refer to main listings.

I

Ibuprofen dosage chart, 20–21
Immunizations
  chicken pox, **75**
  diphtheria, **100**
  German measles, **124**
  measles, **150**
  mumps, **158**
  polio, **171**
  recommended schedule, 8
  record of, 230
  tetanus, **198**
  whooping cough, **210**
Impetigo, **142**
Influenza, **143**, 173
Ingrown toenail, **144**
Injury prevention, 9
Iron
  deficiency, 34
  supplementation, 15
Itching, 39, 46, 75, 108, 166, 167, 178, 193
  throat, 33
  scalp, 129

J

Jaundice, 34, 134, **145**
Joint
  pain, 37, 148, 187
  swelling, 37, 147

L

Laryngitis, **146**
Laxitives, 36, 88
Leg pain, **147**
Lethargy, 110, 151, 173
Leukemia, **148**
Lice
  See Head lice.
Light-headedness, 116, 191
Lips
  blue, 76, 78, 80, 89
  swollen, 33
Liver pain, 134
Lyme disease, 110, **149**

Lymph gland, swollen, 48, 74, 129, 148, 155, 185, **194**

M

Measles, **150**
  See also German measles.
Medicine dosage charts, 19–21
Memory loss, 87
Meningitis, **151**
Menstrual irregularity, **152**
Mole, **153**
  See also Birthmarks.
Molluscum contagiosum, **154**
Mongolian spot, 43
Mononucleosis, **155**
Mood swings, 138
Motion sickness, **156**
Mouth
  and tooth injury, **157**
  blisters in, **67**, 127, 136
  dry, 96
  patches in, 123, 199
  tingling in, 85
Mr. Yuk, 11
Mumps, **158**
Muscle
  aches, 143, 147, 149, 171, 176, 187
  cramps, 133
  spasm, 52, 89, 139, 198

N

Nausea, 33, 36, 45, 87, 101, 122, 125, 131, 133, 134, 156, 170, 182, 197
Neck
  pain, 40
  stiffness, 110, 151, 171
Nephritis, **159**
Nightmares, **160**

Nose
  bleeding, **161**, 162, 163
  injury, **161**, **163**
  object in, **162**
  runny, 33, 84, 100, 124, 128, 146
  stuffy, 128
Numbness, 120, 139
Nutrition, 14–15
  food pyramid, 14

O

Oral health, 16, 202

P

Paleness, 34, 148, 156, 182
Paralysis, 40, 100, 171
Pertussis
  See Whooping cough.
Pierced-ear infection, **164**
Pimple, **30**, **31**, 154, 172
  on eyelid, 190
Pinkeye, **165**
Pinworms, **166**
Pityriasis rosea, **167**
Pneumonia, 95, **168**
Poison ivy, **169**
Poisoning, 11, **170**
Polio, **171**
Port wine stain, 43
Pulse, rapid, 34, 133, 182

R

Rash, 30, 33, 46, 74, 75, 108, 118, 124, 149, 150, 167, 169, 174, 175, 176, 177, 179, 181
  newborn, 31, 91, **98**, **132**, **172**
  See also Diaper rash.
Reye's syndrome, 18, 143, **173**
Rheumatic fever, **174**
Ringworm, **175**

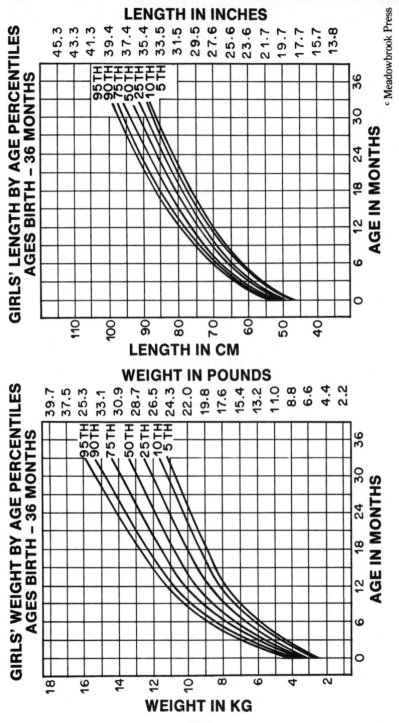

LENGTH IN INCHES

45.3 43.3 41.3 39.4 37.4 35.4 33.5 31.5 29.5 27.6 25.6 23.6 21.7 19.7 17.7 15.7 13.8

GIRLS' LENGTH BY AGE PERCENTILES
AGES BIRTH – 36 MONTHS

95TH
90TH
75TH
50TH
25TH
10TH
5TH

36   30   24   18   12   6   0

AGE IN MONTHS

110   100   90   80   70   60   50   40

LENGTH IN CM

© Meadowbrook Press

WEIGHT IN POUNDS

39.7 37.5 25.3 33.1 30.9 28.7 26.5 24.3 22.0 19.8 17.6 15.4 13.2 11.0 8.8 6.6 4.4 2.2

GIRLS' WEIGHT BY AGE PERCENTILES
AGES BIRTH – 36 MONTHS

95TH
90TH
75TH
50TH
25TH
10TH
5TH

36   30   24   18   12   6   0

AGE IN MONTHS

18   16   14   12   10   8   6   4   2

WEIGHT IN KG

222

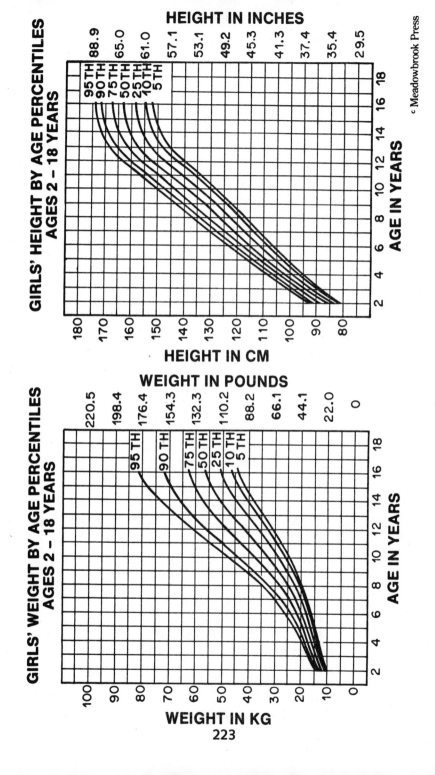

GIRLS' HEIGHT BY AGE PERCENTILES AGES 2 – 18 YEARS

HEIGHT IN INCHES

88.9
65.0
61.0
57.1
53.1
49.2
45.3
41.3
37.4
35.4
29.5

95TH
90TH
75TH
50TH
25TH
10TH
5TH

AGE IN YEARS

HEIGHT IN CM

180
170
160
150
140
130
120
110
100
90
80

c Meadowbrook Press

GIRLS' WEIGHT BY AGE PERCENTILES AGES 2 – 18 YEARS

WEIGHT IN POUNDS

220.5
198.4
176.4
154.3
132.3
110.2
88.2
66.1
44.1
22.0
0

95TH
90TH
75TH
50TH
25TH
10TH
5TH

AGE IN YEARS

WEIGHT IN KG

100
90
80
70
60
50
40
30
20
10
0

223

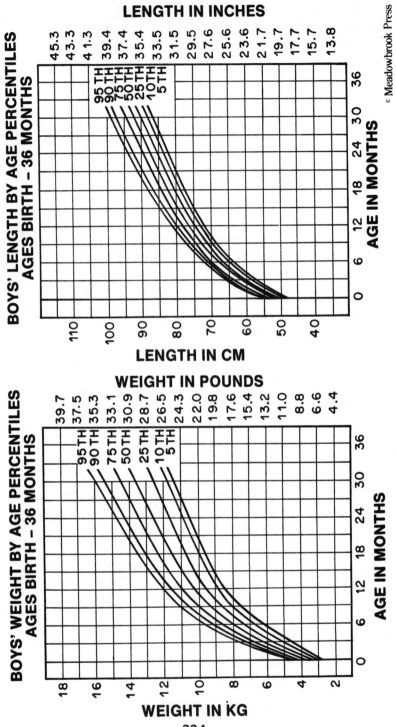

LENGTH IN INCHES

BOYS' LENGTH BY AGE PERCENTILES
AGES BIRTH – 36 MONTHS

45.3 43.3 41.3 39.4 37.4 35.4 33.5 31.5 29.5 27.6 25.6 23.6 21.7 19.7 17.7 15.7 13.8

95 TH
90 TH
75 TH
50 TH
25 TH
10 TH
5 TH

AGE IN MONTHS

0 6 12 18 24 30 36

110 100 90 80 70 60 50 40

LENGTH IN CM

© Meadowbrook Press

WEIGHT IN POUNDS

BOYS' WEIGHT BY AGE PERCENTILES
AGES BIRTH – 36 MONTHS

39.7 37.5 35.3 33.1 30.9 28.7 26.5 24.3 22.0 19.8 17.6 15.4 13.2 11.0 8.8 6.6 4.4

95TH
90TH
75TH
50TH
25TH
10TH
5TH

AGE IN MONTHS

0 6 12 18 24 30 36

18 16 14 12 10 8 6 4 2

WEIGHT IN KG

224

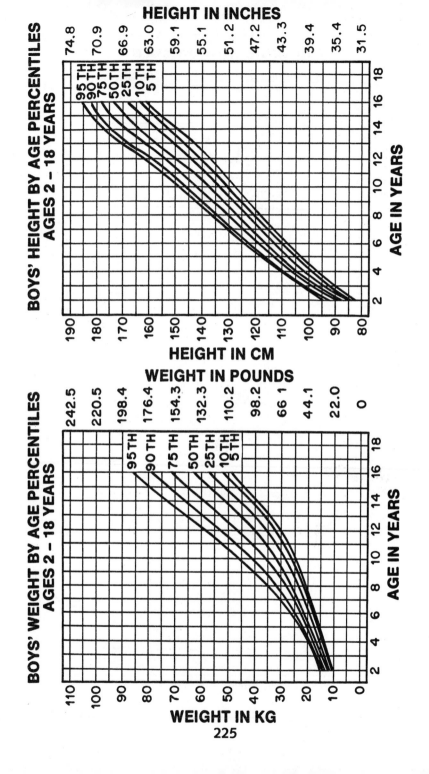

HEIGHT IN INCHES

74.8
70.9
66.9
63.0
59.1
55.1
51.2
47.2
43.3
39.4
35.4
31.5

**BOYS' HEIGHT BY AGE PERCENTILES
AGES 2 – 18 YEARS**

95 TH
90 TH
75 TH
50 TH
25 TH
10 TH
5 TH

AGE IN YEARS

2 4 6 8 10 12 14 16 18

190
180
170
160
150
140
130
120
110
100
90
80

HEIGHT IN CM

WEIGHT IN POUNDS

242.5
220.5
198.4
176.4
154.3
132.3
110.2
98.2
66 1
44.1
22.0
0

**BOYS' WEIGHT BY AGE PERCENTILES
AGES 2 – 18 YEARS**

95TH
90TH
75TH
50TH
25TH
10TH
5TH

AGE IN YEARS

2 4 6 8 10 12 14 16 18

110
100
90
80
70
60
50
40
30
20
10
0

WEIGHT IN KG

225

Immunization Record

For_____	Recommended Age	Date Given	Dosage Preparation	Reaction
1. Hepatitis B-1	2 months			
Hepatitis B-2	4 months			
Hepatitis B-3	6–18 months			
2. DTP (diptheria, tetanus, & pertussis	2 months			
	4 months			
	6 months			
	15–18 months			
	4–6 years			
3. H. influenza type b	2 months			
	4 months			
	6 months			
	12–15 months			
4. Polio	2 months			
	4 months			
	6–18 months			
	4–6 years			
5. MMR (Measles, Mumps, Rubella)	12–15 months			
	4–6 years			
6. Varicella (Chicken Pox)	12–18 months			
7. Tetanus/Diptheria (adult type)	11–16 years			
8. Others				

Photocopy this form for each of your children.

Examinations and Office Calls

For _____

Date	Age	Length/Weight Height	Head Circ. (Infants)	Problems, Diagnoses Laboratory and Other Findings	Doctor's Advice and Comments

Order Form

Qty.	Title	Author	Order No.	Unit Cost (U.S. $)	Total
	15,000+ Baby Names	Lansky, B.	1211	$3.95	
	35,000+ Baby Names	Lansky, B.	1225	$5.95	
	Baby/Child Emergency First Aid	Einzig, M.	1381	$8.00	
	Baby/Child Medical Care	Einzig/Hart	1159	$9.00	
	Baby Name Personality Survey	Lansky, B.	1270	$8.00	
	Best Baby Name Book	Lansky, B.	1029	$5.00	
	Best Baby Shower Book	Cooke, C.	1239	$7.00	
	Best Baby Shower Game Book	Cooke, C.	6063	$3.95	
	Child Care A to Z	Woolfson, R.	1010	$11.00	
	Childhood Medical Record Book	Fix, S.	1130	$10.00	
	Dads Say the Dumbest Things!	Lansky/Jones	4220	$6.00	
	Discipline w/o Shouting/Spanking	Wykoff/Unell	1079	$6.00	
	Familiarity Breeds Children	Lansky, B.	4015	$7.00	
	Feed Me! I'm Yours	Lansky, V.	1109	$9.00	
	First-Year Baby Care	Kelly, P.	1119	$9.00	
	Gentle Discipline	Lighter, D.	1085	$6.00	
	Getting Organized for New Baby	Bard, M.	1229	$9.00	
	Grandma Knows Best	McBride, M.	4009	$7.00	
	How to Read Child Like a Book	Weiss, L.	1145	$8.00	
	Joy of Parenthood	Blaustone, J.	3500	$7.00	
	Moms Say the Funniest Things!	Lansky, B.	4280	$6.00	
	Pregnancy, Childbirth, Newborn	Simkin/Whalley/Keppler	1169	$12.00	
	Very Best Baby Name Book	Lansky, B.	1030	$8.00	
				Subtotal	
			Shipping and Handling (see below)		
			MN residents add 6.5% sales tax		
				Total	

YES! Please send me the books indicated above. Add $2.00 shipping and handling for the first book and 50¢ for each additional book. Add $2.50 to total for books shipped to Canada. Overseas postage will be billed. Allow up to four weeks for delivery. Send check or money order payable to Meadowbrook Press. No cash or C.O.D's please. Prices subject to change without notice. **Quantity discounts available upon request.**

Send book(s) to:

Name _____ Address _____

City _____ State _____ Zip _____

Telephone (_____)_____ P.O. number (if necessary) _____

Payment via:

❑ Check or money order payable to Meadowbrook Press (No cash or C.O.D.'s please)
    Amount enclosed $ _____
❑ Visa (for orders over $10.00 only)   ❑ MasterCard (for orders over $10.00 only)
Account # _____ Signature _____ Exp. Date _____

A _FREE_ Meadowbrook Press catalog is available upon request.
You can also phone us for orders of $10.00 or more at 1-800-338-2232.

Mail to: Meadowbrook Press
5451 Smetana Drive, Minnetonka, MN 55343

Phone (612) 930-1100   Toll -Free 1-800-338-2232   Fax (612) 930-1940